# INKWELL

Simple Writing
Practices to
Restore Your Soul

# INKWELL

ANNE
ELROD
WHITNEY

BROADLEAF BOOKS
MINNEAPOLIS

INKWELL
Simple Writing Practices to Restore Your Soul



Cover image: Shutterstock
Cover design: Olga Grlic

Print ISBN: 978-1-5064-6479-4
eBook ISBN: 978-1-5064-6480-0

# Contents


| | | |
|---|---|---|
| | Acknowledgments | vii |
| **1** | Writing as a Tool for Self-Care | 1 |
| **2** | God's Stories, Our Stories | 11 |
| **3** | Showing Up: Writing for Mindful Presence | 55 |
| **4** | Everyday Discernment | 91 |
| **5** | Writing in Devotion and Prayer | 117 |
| **6** | Write to Survive, Write to Thrive | 141 |
| | Appendix: *Writing with Others: Some Notes for Leaders* | 149 |
| | Notes | 157 |

# Acknowledgments

I wrote most of this book in 2020, which most people will remember as a year like no other. Without guidance from Emily King, I never would have started it, and without astounding grace from Emily and all of the excellent people at Broadleaf Books / 1517 Media, especially Rachel Reyes, I never would have finished it. And without finishing it, I never would have been able to do, again, with full attention, the writing activities in it, which have been so helpful to me through times of growth.

The truth about teaching, about writing, and really about most everything is that we rarely invent from nothing. Many of the writing activities in this book either emulate or adapt things I have learned from others, and I have done my best to properly attribute those ideas but have most certainly failed to acknowledge someone. Most of the best things I know about encouraging groups of writers I learned from Sheridan Blau, my academic father. Any teacher linked to the magnificent network that is the National Writing Project will know almost all of what I am sharing, and they will know also how the best teaching ideas are almost always things we learned from a fellow teacher.

Beyond that, every writing move here has also been developed and revised with specific audiences in mind: the people who have gathered with me in writing groups, retreats, and workshops. Among these are special friends who sent me examples of writing they had done at home, even consenting to have them included in the book (and while they ultimately were not, the hearts and lives of these friends are on every page: Ellen Campbell, Shelbie Witte, Cathy Fleischer, Jayne Steff, Phoebe Quaynor, Libby Snyder, Boni Richardson, Linda Giles, Cheryl Hogue Smith, Linda Andrews, Nicole Damico, Usep Syaripudin, and Yen Yun-Chen). Alicia Anderson of Penn State Lutheran Campus Ministry and Nathan and Angie Pile of Camp Sequanota were especially generous in inviting me to lead retreats, as well as State College Presbyterian Church and Grace Lutheran Church, especially Dotty Delafield. Two other heroes, Lois Lynn and Steve Lynn, read and responded to almost the entire manuscript, sharing their writing and insights as freely as they have shared their many gifts in the fifteen years I have known them. Steve may recognize a couple of shared moments here too.

# 1

# WRITING AS A TOOL FOR SELF-CARE

"Take care!"

It's an expression, just a way we sometimes say goodbye. It's right there on the small talk shelf, next to "How are you?" and "I'm fine": one of those nice-but-empty statements that I hear and say without thinking.

But a few years ago, I suddenly couldn't hear that little phrase "take care" without thinking in reply, *I already am*.

I was taking care of a family. Of cooking and cleaning and organizing and scheduling and tidying. I was taking care of dentist appointments and dropping off the forgotten clarinet and getting more toilet paper and reminding everyone to wash their hands and brush their teeth. Of shoveling the sidewalk, and knowing everyone's clothing sizes, and mailing out Christmas cards, and finding black shoes for the concert that's tonight. Of nurse phone calls and visits from the plumber. I was taking care of hot tempers and adolescent changes and mean kids on the playground and boring homework.

And I was taking care of a career. Of email and reports and recommendations and schedules. Of research projects and doctoral students and committee meetings and evaluations. Of travel and presentations, articles and book contracts. I was taking care of colleagues and bringing cake to the faculty meeting and mentoring and leading meetings and unjamming the printer.

"I don't know how you do it," people in my life would say. "You make it look easy." But however it looked, it was *not* easy.

I was taking care of details, taking care of business.

I was not taking care of *myself.*

I slept poorly. I had higher anxiety, blood pressure, weight, stress, and irritability than normal. I had a lower mood, energy, productivity, and joy than normal. I felt all-around less *normal* than normal. I cried on the daily, slept rarely, and fumed mightily at all manner of wrongs. I prayed less, sang less, loved less, yelled more, hurt more, complained more. I was not OK. And being not-OK was becoming a way of life rather than something I went through every now and then.

You care for your car, for your houseplants, for your body, and for your money. What about your self? Your spiritual self? To function and thrive as the spiritual beings that we are, we need care just as much.

## WHY SELF-CARE?

On the personal scale, many of us are stressed and overwhelmed: We are living in a time and place in which busyness is seen as a sign of importance. Devices keep us in a tension between constant connection and disconnection: We are constantly reachable and aware of others online, while at the same time, that availability interrupts our connection to those with whom we are physically present. Even children are overstretched across a variety of resume-building activities. This is not good for us.

On the larger scale, we are hurting too: Issues of inequity seem intractable. Racism, sexism, homophobia, xenophobia, economic oppression, violence both physical and spiritual: these issues persist and even worsen, and for those who dedicate themselves to activism or change, the work is often discouraging. Those who give care know this to be true: teachers, faith leaders, health care workers, and others in helping roles struggle with burnout at alarming rates. But this struggle is not limited to those whose profession involves care: all sorts of people, from students to parents to everyday people of faith, find themselves needing a break from the news or from engaging the issues they find important, with a feeling that the problems are just too far gone by now.

We need practices that deliberately reorient us amid these challenges—practices that reconnect our attention to God, to the world around us, to other people, and to ourselves. (I'll say more about God, as well as how to use this book regardless of your belief or unbelief, in chapter 2.)

Sometimes I hear people saying that an organization, leader, or experience "didn't feed them." I know what that means, and I have had disappointing spiritual experiences too. But ultimately, we are not dependent on others for spiritual health, though others can be supports, guides, and companions, and organizations can provide conditions for spiritual health. We can rely on God to care for our spirits, and we can engage in God's action by taking responsibility for self-care. It's like the old joke: A person says, "God will save me" from an impending disaster, and thus stands motionless, "relying on God" when meanwhile, God is sending a rowboat, a helicopter, a team of rescuers, and more, all of which the person ignores. The sun feeds the plants, but that doesn't mean we shouldn't still weed the garden. Spiritual self-care requires attention on our part. We can, and must, feed ourselves.

## WHY WRITING?

Writing offers particular benefits for self-care. First, when writing, we stop time, however briefly. Writing can only be undertaken mindfully, keeping us attached to the moment that we are actually in. Consider how you can drive home from work and pull into your driveway without realizing how you made the trip. Think of how you can read several pages in a book and then look up, finding that you don't really know what you have read even though your eyes and brain decoded every word. Writing is different from this in that it is impossible to do it automatically: When you write, you have to keep both your body and your mind engaged. When your mind wanders, your pen stops moving or your fingers stop typing. When we write, we can't be projecting too far into the future or into the past. Yes, we can be writing about past events or about future imaginings, but in doing so, we remain rooted in the perspective of *right now*. This mindful state is one that many faith traditions and wellness modalities have used for spiritual awareness and growth.[1,2,3]

Second, research reveals many therapeutic benefits of writing, from physiological to psychological to relational. Best known among scholars of these therapeutic qualities of writing is James Pennebaker, a psychology researcher at the University of Texas at Austin. Since the 1980s, he and his colleagues have investigated writing as a therapeutic tool. The first experiments involved inviting randomly selected people (usually college students, who are readily available and usually willing to participate in studies in exchange for a few extra credit points) to enter a room, write for twenty minutes, and then leave, depositing their writing in a box on their way out. After doing this for a few weeks, these students showed a range of effects as compared to a control group: They reported better moods, scored lower on measures of depression and anxiety, took fewer days off work or from classes due to illness, visited the health center less often, and even had lower resting heart rates and blood pressure. These effects varied according to the writing prompt used and the frequency and duration of the writing practice, but the overall finding is now established through a subsequent thirty years of research: Writing is beneficial as a practice, on its own, outside of any transaction in which an audience reads the writing or even whether the writers themselves ever read back over it. It's not the text written that matters so much as the activity of writing, inclusive of its physical, mental, emotional, and spiritual components.[4,5,6,7,8]

Third, writing is free and accessible. You don't need special supplies, or to travel to a special location, or to have any special skills beyond the basic literacy you are using to read this book. Writing's benefits accrue to any writer, regardless of experience or skill.

Many of us have had the experience of receiving as a gift a beautiful journal, or of purchasing a journal with grand intentions of establishing a system of writing. This might be at the new year, or as a practice for a particular season (such as Lent for many Christians), or on the occasion of an important life experience such as a trip or the birth of a child or the beginning of something new. Yet in these situations, it's easy to get hung up on doing it "right," for example, by writing beautiful vignettes in a travelogue, or by recounting our family stories in a way that we hope our grandchildren will want to read and treasure. That's a lot of pressure! Or we wait to write—however, the "right time" to write never presents itself. Or it feels like we need the perfect physical context for writing: complete silence, a comfortable chair with a special candle burning, or a fancy pen. Of course, these times and contexts never materialize, and the journal lies empty. Or we get hung up on how the writing will look (my handwriting is too messy; I should type it and then recopy it) or sound (I don't have the right words; I've been away from school for too long; I've never been an "English person"), and we find ourselves too intimidated to begin. If we've had these experiences, we may even have added a layer of shame on the top for ourselves: When I studied the writing practices of Christian pastors, for example, I asked, "Do you use a journal or notebook?" The most common answer was a lowered head, a rueful look, and the words, "I know I should . . ." None of these lines of thinking offer benefit of any kind! I know I'm great at making myself feel horrible just by tuning into the radio stations that play in my head. I don't need help feeling bad from another "should-do" that I don't get around to. In this book, we will work to replace beliefs about writing that hurt us with writing habits that are self-compassionate, flexible, and realistic.

## IN THIS BOOK: WRITING AS SPIRITUAL REFLECTION FOR ACTION

We tend to have experiences and then quickly move to the next without processing what has happened. This means that we miss out on opportunities to learn from—or even to notice!—what we experience. That which goes unnoticed and unthought about is basically lost to us. If it's something good, we miss out. If it's something bad, that something may keep happening again and again. I compare this to dating: Most of us, by the time we are adults, have had a few relationships that didn't work out. And for many of us, we eventually look back and realize that all those partners were similar, or that our own actions within the relationships repeatedly undermined us. If we never reflect on our experiences, how are we to learn from them?

Reflection turns experiences into learning—it makes them our own.[9] While we often hear words like "I'll reflect on that," what does reflection really mean? It's something we tend to agree is good to do, but we're not specific enough about what it means. Reflection isn't just thinking about something; thinking could be ruminating, recalling, solving, meditating, or any of a number of other cognitive processes. No, I've learned that reflection is actually pretty specific. From its Latin roots, to reflect is to "re-," as in "again," and it is to "-flect," as in "bend," or "turn," -flect as in "flexible." So to reflect on something includes to think flexibly about it, to bend it around in new ways, or turn it and see it from new angles or perspectives. And the truth about reflection is that we don't necessarily do it easily. Reflecting, seeing something from a new angle or returning to something to follow it around a new bend, can be challenging. It can require that we change our minds, or it can break understandings of the world that we thought were working for us. Like any learning, reflection means that sometimes we lose something we thought we knew.

In this book, we will write to *reflect* through reflection's three components: *remember, describe, act*. These three components have a backstory: When I worked with second- and third-grade teachers who were helping their students with reflection,[10] I realized that just saying, "OK, now reflect on what you've just done" isn't really enough direction. Together, through experimentation and close observation of kids, we learned that kids needed to do at least three basic moves in order to reflect meaningfully. First, they had to remember what they had done in the first place. Maybe it sounds obvious, but the truth is most seven- and eight-year-olds may not remember what they had for breakfast one morning, much less something more significant, without a little help. Like the kids, our own memories need a little prompting too. Maybe we recall an important event, but what more about it can we recall? What was said? What was the weather like? What happened first, second, third, and so on? Those additional details can help us to understand the memory in a different way.

Second, reflection also involves describing what we remember. That is, reflection happens through language, and the more specific language we can find to put on our experiences, the more we can also refine, revise, and/or rewrite the meanings of those experiences. For instance, when we wanted the second and third graders to reflect on experiences in the writing classroom, they were helped by learning specific vocabulary for writing, words like "edit" and "emphasis" and "elaborate" and "imagery." Instead of saying, "my story got better," they could say, "in the first draft, I told the story, but then I revised to include more vivid imagery." Putting words onto an experience helps us move from simply being a character in the story to being its author or coauthor. What we can describe, we can also interpret.

Third, reflection includes attention to action. Once we come to see something in a new way, or with greater clarity, or with new connections, we're bound to live out those realizations. Whether it is direct action like going out and joining a gym, ending a relationship, and so on or whether it's a more subtle action like resolving to establish better boundaries with coworkers in the future, or praying more wholeheartedly, or taking a more open-minded stance toward a certain person, reflection is tied to action. We can use writing to name, plan, and even track outcomes of our actions.

All of these reflective moves, from remembering to describing to acting, help us care for ourselves. The spiritual self-care that writing can provoke is much like what you would do for a friend needing spiritual support: You would listen to that person carefully, you would remember what they said, and you would link it to things you knew about that person or their situation from past experiences too. The person and their problem would have your attention, perhaps the greatest gift we can give another person (or ourselves). You would work, either aloud with that friend or in your own heart, for understanding and empathy to describe what's really going on, as in "She's sad about the date being canceled, but I see she's also scared of ending up alone," or "He's discouraged. He's wondering whether he matters." And while it helps that friend just to be heard (and maybe sticking around to hear more is itself a form of action), you might also do more: Hug her. Bring brownies. Forgive her for snapping at you. Invite him somewhere. Give him time. Actions like these, caring actions we might take for a friend, are actions we deserve for ourselves just as much—and writing will help us to identity and take appropriate actions for ourselves.

## HOW TO USE THIS BOOK

The main way to use this book is: Write in it. I don't mean that in a snarky way; what I am saying is that, like an exercise program, or practicing the piano, or building any new skill or habit, nothing will happen if you never actually do it. Get a pen, whether it's a fancy one or a chewed-up, free one you accidentally stole from the bank. Sit somewhere, whether it's in a peaceful writing corner or the break room on your lunch hour or in the car outside of your kid's dancing school or in your kitchen, at a quiet time or a noisy time. And then try doing what the book suggests.

I hope it goes without saying by this point that it doesn't matter if you stop for a while. You can start up again, with no need to start over. Pick up where you left off.

The ideas in this book will be most helpful if you simply try them, with as little self-editing or judgment as you can. You're not creating a record for posterity, and nobody will even see what you write unless you make a choice to share it. The audience is you, and some of the content not even *you* will read again. Try not to care about all those things that usually slow writers down. Don't worry about sounding smart, or spelling things correctly, or your handwriting. Forget whether what you're writing is "right" or "good" or even true—just write what comes to mind in response to the prompts along the way. Trust that this time you spend with yourself, writing, is time well spent. Even your presence, being there for yourself enough to make the effort to write, is a way of saying to your own soul, "You matter. I'm paying attention."

# 2

# GOD'S STORIES, OUR STORIES

We are story people. Stories are our entertainment. They are how we get to know one another. They are how we escape, or how we make sense. Our holy texts are made primarily from stories. They are how we tell each other—and ourselves—who we are.

It makes sense, then, to start with stories. In this chapter, we will use writing to explore how our stories show us ourselves, and how they show us God's presence in our lives. We'll explore different kinds of stories. For each, you'll find invitations to *draw or jot*, to *write*, and to *reread and reflect* on what you've written.

A note about God: this book is for people of any faith, including people of no faith. My own tradition is a Christian one, and when I say God, it means something specific to me. I will name specifically some particulars of my own faith life as a Christian of the Lutheran variety, within the church widely as well as specific churches and congregations. And I will name the divine as God, as Jesus, as the Holy Spirit. But your divine and my divine do not have to match. For the purposes of this book, God can mean whatever makes most sense for you: the divine as expressed in your faith tradition, the divine as you imagine or experience it, or even like some twelve-step community members understand it: the collective power of a human community.

## WRITING AND READING OUR FAITH STORIES

Stories help us process, understand, and communicate about what happens in our lives. Have you ever been in a car accident? At first, when you try to recount what happened, the details come out jumbled, in a kind of flood of information. However, as you tell the story again and again to your family, to the doctor, to the police, to your employer, you get better at telling it. The story becomes more and more neatly packaged as you figure out what's important and what can be omitted, which details need to be explained as exposition before you get to the moment of impact, and what order of explanation makes most sense to your listeners. By telling the story, we get better at packaging it, bringing out key themes.

Faith stories are like this too. Through writing and rewriting stories of our faith lives, we benefit in several ways. One is that we come to new understandings about what we have been through. We come to see what we thought we knew about a time in life or about a significant experience differently after time has passed, or when viewed through a different lens. This is what it means to grow.

Another benefit, and one no less important, is that as we shape and curate stories, we also are better prepared to share them. Sharing stories about our lives strengthens our connections to one another. Sharing stories about our faith lives strengthens our connections to members of our faith communities—but it is also, of course, how we bear witness to what God has done. Think of the women who first told how they had found the tomb of Jesus, opened, and then had found Jesus himself, alive! What if they hadn't told?

A third benefit is that writing our stories gives us power over them: the power of revision. No, you can't exactly change what has happened like you might in a piece of fiction, but you can revise in other ways. Like a manuscript of a poem or a short story, your stories can be revised to bring out different details, to add complexity, or to weave in counternarratives. You can emphasize a different theme, reinterpret, or even manipulate the point of view. In these ways, we review and revise stories that have controlled us in the past, taking control of their meanings going forward.

## My Stories with God

### Draw

I know it's a little ironic that a book about writing will start with a bit of drawing. But that's exactly where I'd like to start.

Get a pen or a pencil: preferably something stubby with no eraser, or maybe a free pen from a hotel or a conference you attended with the cap chewed off by one of your kids on a particularly tough homework night. Or it can be your favorite pen too, if it's nearby and it doesn't make you picky about what your writing looks like. You want to use the most basic, unintimidating materials possible, because you are about to draw a very bad drawing.

Now, I'd like you to map,[1] or draw—not write—your story with God. When I do this with groups, I set a timer for five to ten minutes, and you might like to do the same. With that tiny amount of time, there's no chance you will make a good-looking map—and that's the point. Some people will draw a map like a map of land. Make it a rough and ugly map, as though you're giving driving directions to someone (back in the olden days when we gave directions, before we all had maps built into our phones). Others will draw a sort of graph, with a midline stretching horizontally across the paper representing medium or neutral times, then graphing a timeline with high points shooting up above the midline and low points dipping down below the midline as time passes. Other people will depict a winding path or road, with interesting stops on their journey marked on the side of the path as they go. Other people seize on a focal image, like a cloud, or a tornado, or a mountain, or a house. It really doesn't matter. Please don't think too hard about this. Don't make a good drawing. Don't create a work of art. You won't be showing it to anyone. Instead, just set your timer (or just the timer in your head) for about four minutes and do a bit of sketching. What has your journey with God been like? What have some of the important waypoints been? What have some strong points been, and what have been some misfortunes along the way? What was God doing at this time or at that time?

Once you've got your map, the next thing is to spend time marking some story places on that map. I like to use stars and then label the spot or sometimes even title the story, just so I can come back to it later on. For example, one spot on my own map is Camp Lone Star. I might just draw a hill with a cross on it and jot "Lone Star" there so I don't forget. I have some important stories that happened there. Another one might be the parking lot where I packed up my car to drive out of Texas, to what was truly a contiguous state (New Mexico) but may as well have been a world away from the Houston suburbs where I grew up. I didn't know then that I

✍

wouldn't be coming back to Houston, or even Texas, again. Or, there's a story place where I entered a church after many years away. There's a story place where I listened to the Christian radio from my bedroom in middle school, in Houston in the 1980s, wanting to know more about God and wondering where God was in all of the radio talk about Sin and Abomination and, what seemed to me weirdest of all, the End Times. There's a story place in my high school yearbook and it's pictures of me doing activities mostly with a smile on my face, but no pictures of the times I sat alone, or hid in my car rather than going to a class, or just called in and stayed home because I couldn't make myself go to school. There's a story place in the birth of my first child, and the way that after she was born, every single adult looked to me like a former baby.

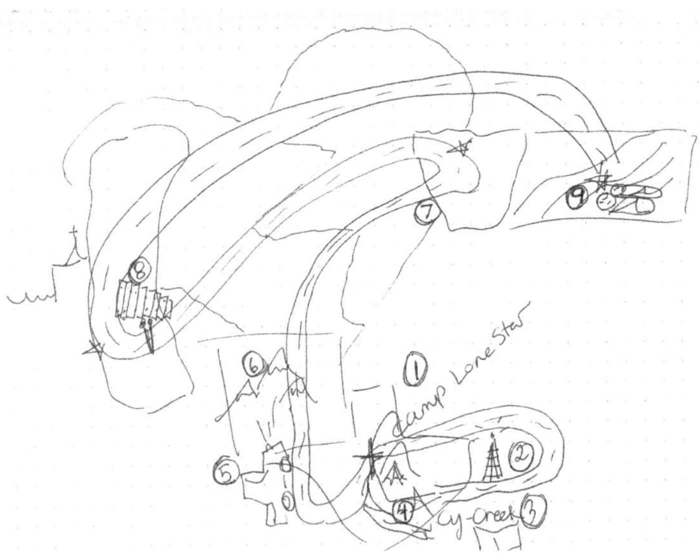


All of these places fit together into a giant map of a life story. Depending on who we're talking to at a given moment, we might pick up any one or two or three of those small stories to tell as part of the larger one. At this point, it doesn't really matter which one you pick. Look back over your map and see if there are one or two story places that stand out to you as important as to how you see your story with God. Maybe one is a story you haven't thought about in a very long time. Maybe one is a story you've thought about (or even told) a lot, but you never really thought of it as being a story about God. Maybe one is about a time you felt especially close to God. Or one is about a time you had no idea whether God was even there. Number your story places now.

Once you've marked and numbered some story places, can you think about titles for some of the stories? I've listed mine here:

(1) From "Nothing" to Everything
(2) Waiting for your Call
(3) I'll Just Be In My Car, Reading
(4) Long, Long, Gone and Gone
(5) Following, Following, Desert Paths
(6) Holy Crap (This Is What They Were Talking About)
(7) Wait, was that Even who I Was?
(8) Priestly Vibes
(9) Once a Baby . . .

Don't overthink these titles, but do try to name each story. Don't worry, you're not committing to writing all of these; you're just thinking about what they'd be called if they were little short stories, or movies, or episodes of a TV show.

1. ______________________________
2. ______________________________
3. ______________________________
4. ______________________________
5. ______________________________
6. ______________________________
7. ______________________________
8. ______________________________
9. ______________________________
10. ______________________________

### Jot

Pick one of these stories and think about it for a minute. Then, take a moment just to list some words. These are sensory words. What did you see at that time? What did you hear at that time—what words were people saying, or what sounds were in the environment then? What smells were about? What tastes? How did your body feel? All you need here is a list of sensory words that put you back in the story for just a moment. Thinking about Camp Lone Star, the first place and time that I ever talked about God out loud at all, I remember the deep itch of chigger bites. Nothing else itches quite like those. I remember the sounds of hearty campfire singing, complete with harmonies, the first I'd ever tried to sing myself. I remember dining hall mashed potatoes, the first I'd ever eaten (as a picky eater, I'd never quite been hungry enough before to try them, but a day of camp makes a kid very hungry). I remember the sound of a rifle at skeet shooting; I remember the taste of a frozen 100 Grand bar I purchased from the camp Trading Post. I remember the sound of locusts and crickets and all the other bug sounds of the Texas hill country in the summer. I remember heat, scorching heat; sweaty skin; cool popsicles; the shock of slightly frozen Nehi orange soda in a glass bottle from an old-timey soda machine.

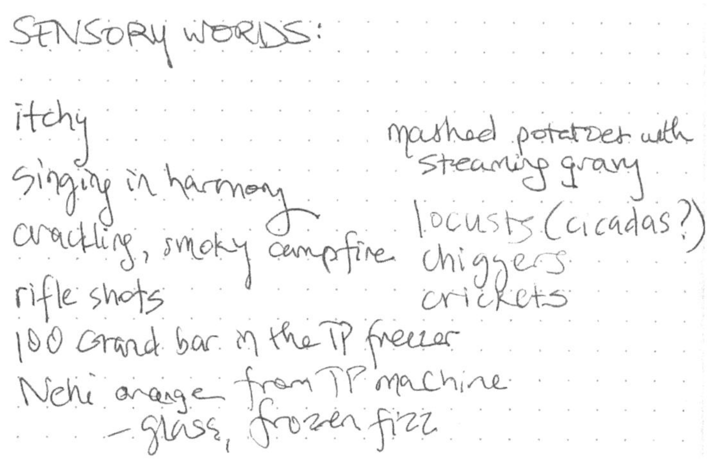

### Write

Once you've got these words, set a timer for seven minutes. I just use the one on my phone. My academic mentor, who has led a lot of writing workshops with a lot of adults, likes to say that seven minutes is about a unit of adult thought. I think he's right. Almost any time I do a workshop where there's quick writing, or journaling, or writing to debrief after an activity, seven minutes is about the right amount of time. Enough time for a thought, but not enough time to dwell on the thought, or to worry if it's a good thought, or to really finish writing it down. It's just enough to get started and to develop a thought enough to write something. You want to keep going for at least seven minutes. You'll often find you want to go much more than that—go ahead! (On my own, my seven minutes tends to turn into fifteen.) But seven minutes is a good target; it's enough.

Now, for seven minutes or so, simply quickwrite the story you've been remembering. Don't worry about spelling well, or crafting a lovely narrative, or presenting the story in any particular way. Don't worry about how it sounds at all. Just write, as much as you can, as quickly as you can. Some teachers call this "Fast and Furious" writing, though you need not be furious or even particularly fast. Many writers and teachers also call this "word vomit," which is disgusting but makes the point that what you need to be is unselfconscious. Just brain-dump. Just get it down in the most basic way that you can. You're not really making anything; you're simply collecting information at this point. Write for seven minutes. Don't stop. Just keep going for seven minutes.

When the seven minutes are up, you've got a story, or at least the beginning of one. If there are things you meant to get to but didn't have time for, write a few notes to yourself about those at the bottom. Maybe you'll finish later. Maybe you won't. (Maybe you'll just set the timer for another seven right now, or just write without any timer at all.) It doesn't matter at this point. You're writing for the experience of writing about it, for what you might notice along the way, for what your own writing might show you. You're not writing in order to make anything for any other person. So it doesn't matter if you're not done—but you might want to make a few notes just so that whatever your brain cooks up isn't forgotten. My brain forgets fast.

✍

✍

## Read and Reflect

We're writing not only for the sake of the writing itself but also for what we can learn from the process. So, let's take a few minutes to look back over what you have written. Throughout this book, I'll share a variety of strategies for rereading, analyzing, and learning from what you've written. Once you get the idea, you'll be able to mix and match these on your own.

*What is the story about?*

The first thing I like to do is simply read back what I have written, with all of my curiosity turned up to maximum. I try to read the story as though it were written by someone else. I'm not reading it to evaluate, to decide whether it's a good writing or anything, but simply reading with the question: What is this story about?[2] The power of that question—what is this story about?—is that this writing might have more than one meaning. It could have meanings that you as its author put in purposely, but it could also have other meanings that you hadn't noticed or thought about when you were writing it. Read over your writing, wondering, "what is the story about?" Sometimes it's helpful to jot a list of *possible* things it could be about. Don't worry, you're not committing to anything; the point is just to generate some possibilities. For example, my story about Camp Lone Star could be about newfound independence, traveling away from family for the first time. It could be about the witness of God's grace through the other people who welcomed me at camp and made me feel at home. It could be a story about friendships, developed away from school and its cliques and pressure, for a girl who often felt left out. It could be a story about being in nature in which, in the hills and vistas of an especially gorgeous part of Texas,

I found also a different perspective on God and on life. What might your story be about? Make some jottings.

✍

*Golden lines*

Another thing to try with what you've written is to read over it, searching for one or two "golden lines."[3] A golden line is one of those lines that when you read it, you're a bit surprised you wrote it. Maybe it stands out because you like how it sounds. Maybe it's one of those lines that's just so *true* that it's like a bell ringing, its sound slicing through the rest with its sudden honesty. Maybe it's a golden line because it captures so precisely a feeling or an image. Maybe you just like it a lot. Read through your writing above, under "Write," and underline or circle one or more golden lines.

Try copying one of those golden lines at the top of the writing space below. You could spend another seven minutes quickwriting about it. What comes up that didn't come up before? What do you notice now? This is a powerful strategy for getting to the bottom of things. Write something, reread it, grab a golden line, write again off of that line, repeat.

✍

## My Stories with the Church

There's your relationship with God, and then there's your relationship with the church. Sometimes these are hand-in-hand, working together harmoniously like two voices in the same song. Other times they're in conflict. It can be really useful to spend some time reflecting upon your relationship with the church over time. Maybe you were born and raised in the congregation you still attend now. Maybe you were raised in a congregation but left as a teenager and never came back. Maybe you're like me and have moved around the country a lot, trying different churches along the way, with some years of strong involvement and other years avoiding church completely. Maybe something bad happened to you in the church and you walked away from it. Or maybe something bad is happening now. Maybe you're a pastor serving a congregation. Maybe a church community hurt you, or helped you. Maybe you've avoided church, or lost interest, or maybe you serve it and work to shape it. Maybe it excluded you, or maybe it's a home to you. Whatever your particulars, you and the church have stories.

And, maybe you've never been a "church person." That, too, is a relationship with the church, isn't it? These writings aren't one-size-fits-all; reshape them to fit what works for you. "The church" could mean all of organized religion, all institutions connected to one particular faith, or to one particular human organization such as a Christian denomination. It can be a particular congregation, or a group of religious people who have affected you. "Church" here means what you need it to mean in order for the writing to take you somewhere you want to explore.

Many times, we conflate the story of God with the story of the church. They're not quite the same. God is God, and the church is God's, but really the church is us. There's a difference. Writing stories *both* of God, as above, *and* of the church, as we will try below, can help us discern those nuances.

### Draw and/or Jot

Take a few minutes to do some drawing and/or while you think about your history with the church. For some folks, this might be a map of the United States, with different churches you've attended in different places over the years marked on the map. For some people it might be a picture of the one and only building, the church in which you were raised or one you attend now. Maybe it's a sketch of the outside of a church building, or maybe it's a map of the building, from a bird's-eye view. Maybe it's a few quick images of things you remember from churches that have been important to you (in positive ways, negative ways, or any ways in between), like a particular cross, or window, or font, or kitchen, or parking lot. And of course it's not only the building; the church is the people. Maybe specific pastors or church members or musicians have meant a lot to you. What songs have been important? What sounds? What physical sensations? What foods—covered dishes? Beans and rice? Easter candy? Communion wafers or crusty homemade bread? Scorched coffee?

Again, the idea here is not to make a lovely picture, or to produce any complete record of anything. It's to gather up some building materials that you'll use later in your writing. A map can help you remember. Some sensory words can put you back in the scene. Thinking about the church as a place is only one way of thinking about it, but it can be provocative. It's just a building, but a lot of important things may have

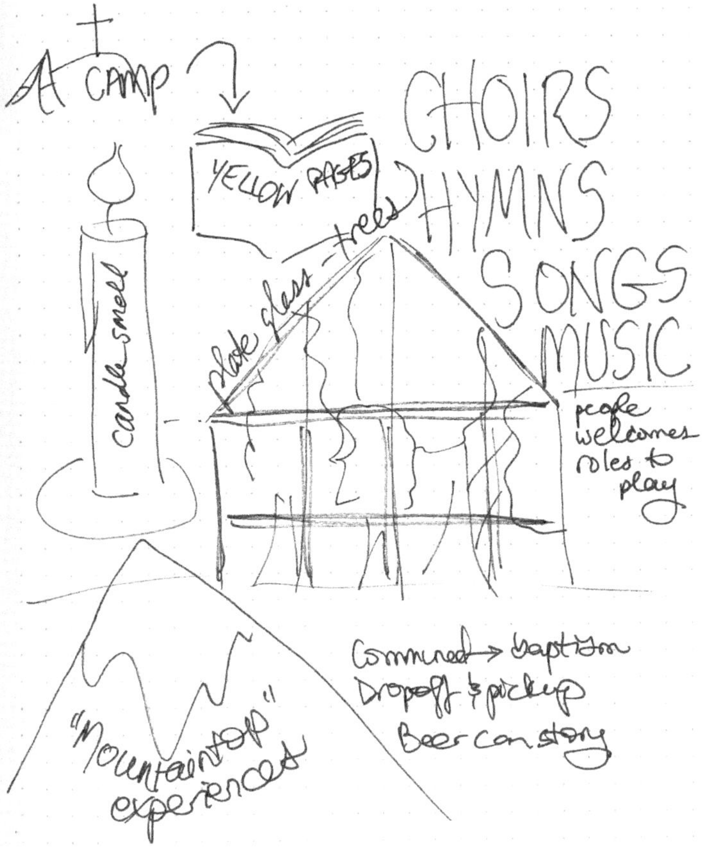
CAMP
YELLOW PAGES
CHOIRS
HYMNS
SONGS
MUSIC
trees
plate glass
candle smell
people welcomes roles to play
Communed → baptism
Dropoff & pickup
Beer can story
"Mountaintop" experience

happened inside that building. Maybe your story with the church involves educational institutions, like a grade school, a college, or a seminary. Maybe it's a story about books you've read, from the children's Bible you had as a child to C. S. Lewis when you were a teenager. I don't know; our stories are as varied as our lives. Make some drawings; jot some one- or two-word notes. What have been some important places, people, text, objects, and times in your life in the church?

Once you've got some drawings, or some jottings, spend a few moments simply remembering. I like to place my finger on the paper and touch different parts of the map or my notes. As I do that, some images or ideas simply jump out more than others. If this happens for you, mark a couple of those with stars, or with a highlighter.

### Write

When you're ready, do some brain-dump-type writing about your story with the church. Don't spend time worrying about choosing the right story or the right starting point; anywhere is the right place. Maybe it's a particular congregation, where something changed in your relationship with God through that. Maybe it's a time the church disappointed you, and you want to say those words out loud (or at least write them out loud) once and for all. You don't have to choose the most important story or the best story; all you need to do right now is choose a story and start writing it, as quickly and nonjudgmentally as you can.

Here are some ideas that may get you writing. Don't try to tackle all of these at once. Just grab one for now and know that you can come back to the list again and again:

What is your earliest church memory?

What was your experience with church as a child? How, if at all, has that changed as you've grown up and aged?

What's your story with church music? Do particular hymns or songs provoke particular memories?

With whom have you sat in worship over the years? Who sits with you now? Or do you sit on your own?

When has the church made you proud to be a Christian? When has it embarrassed you?

When has the church disappointed you or caused you difficulty?

When has the church helped you through something difficult?

Who first took you to church, or invited you to try it? What did you expect, and how did the experience meet or defy your expectations?

What do you love in a worship service? What makes you cringe?

Did you ever cry in worship? What happened?

What words from worship do you know by heart? What have those meant to you? Have those meanings changed with time?

Have you spent time without a worshipping community, or are you without one now? How did that come to be? How does it feel?

What's your story with the Bible (or another holy text from your own tradition)? Is it a book you've read cover to cover? One you've dipped into from time to time? When has Scripture comforted you, and when has it hurt you? Are there words you come back to again and again?

Is there a story about your experience with the Bible or another holy text from your own tradition as a physical object? What does your Bible/book look like—is it worn, with a cracked spine and many pencil markings? Was it a gift from someone you love? Do you have shelves of many Bibles, in search of the right translation, or use different editions for different purposes?

How has the church influenced an important relationship? For example, if you're a parent, how has church played a role in the development of your family or your children? If you have or had a significant other, how does your story with church involve or exclude that person? Did that person bring you to church, attend with you, stay away, lead?

Again, the point with this writing is not really to compose a text to be shared, unless you feel moved to share it or are working with a group through this book. And if you do share, the point of the sharing isn't to get an evaluation of the writing or to prove you're a good Christian or a good person. It's simply to bear witness to your own experience.

✍

This idea, of bearing witness, is at the heart of all the informal writing we are doing in this book. Our stories have shaped us, and by writing and reflecting upon them, we also shape ourselves. Often there is power simply in saying out loud or on paper, "this happened to me." Things happened, and you're still here. Things happened, and you responded, or survived, or adapted, or learned, or were grateful or hurt or blessed.

What's more, these stories can help us see where God was at work—and, sometimes, where what we experienced was more about other people than about God. By writing stories about you and the church, you can get to the bottom of this blessed, flawed, beautiful, torn, complicated community we're in of God's people. It's no more perfect than any one of its members—yet like each of its members, along with its brokenness it also has capacity to reflect God's love and grace.

## Read and Reflect

You can reflect on what you've written right away, or you can let some time pass and come back to it. You've already tried two ways of revisiting your writing, earlier in this chapter: asking "What is this story about?" and identifying "golden lines." Here are other ways of digging into what you have written.

### *Verbs I do / verbs God does*

A pastor friend, Mike Price, told me about an exercise he sometimes does with a passage of Scripture. He looks through the passage and makes a list of all the verbs God does. Almost any passage of the Bible reveals a remarkable list if you try this. For example, here's my list from the first fourteen verses of Psalm 103:

forgives
heals
redeems
crowns
satisfies
works vindication
works justice
makes his ways known
removes transgressions
has compassion
knows
remembers

Try this with your own writing. Try using a t-chart: one column lists verbs God does, and the other lists verbs you do. Now, not every verb will be vivid and meaningful, especially since this is quick, unrevised writing. You can expect to see lots of "to be" verbs on your list. These verbs, like "is," "are," and "was," are hardworking but boring on their own; that is, they don't denote striking actions on their own but instead simply point to other parts of a sentence. The verbs you'll learn most from are the vivid action verbs, not these. But still, what does this list help you to notice?

| Verbs God Does | Verbs I Do |
| --- | --- |
| | |

| What does this chart of verbs help you to notice? |
| --- |
| |

*What has come of this?*

Another provocative way of reflecting on what you've written is to ask a simple question: "What has come of this?" Read back over a story of you and the church. For each major event or turn in the story, pause and ask yourself, "What has come of this?" Take a moment to write down what comes to mind.

For example, one of my own stories involves a time when I, as a twelve-year-old junior high school student, showed up for a rehearsal of a folk ensemble that met at the church I had recently started attending. This is a church I had found using the Yellow Pages, picking a Lutheran church after having had a fun week at a Lutheran camp I had attended with my friend. I had come to worship maybe three or four times, my parents dropping me off in the parking lot before driving on home to resume drinking coffee and reading the paper. During worship, I voraciously read through the bulletin, announcements pages, and even the front and back matter of our hymnal, things like indexes and explanations of the order of worship. It was like I had arrived in a foreign land, and I was doing my best to figure out what everything was and how it worked.

In the bulletin, listed on the weekly schedule, I saw the musical ensembles: Adult Choir, Wednesdays at seven, and underneath that, Kairos Folk Ensemble, Thursdays at six thirty. I loved music, choir being a newfound love after I chanced upon the sixth-grade music class. So, a week or two later, I showed up, walking into the small music room down the hallway of the church office wing. There were three or four adults in a semicircle, and some instruments: a guitar, a tambourine, a hammered dulcimer. I am now absolutely certain they did not expect a child to walk in. This was not a youth choir, and no youth had ever tried to join before. But there I was. I showed up wanting to join in some folk music. I don't think I even knew what that meant, but it was music and I was curious. So, they did what I now think was a brave act of welcome. They smiled, gestured toward a chair, and handed me a book! From then on, I was a member of Kairos—even though I often didn't come to rehearsal if I couldn't get a ride, or if I just forgot, and I had nothing like the musical skills of the adult members. Those people so welcomed me that it was only years later, as an adult, that I actually realized it was out of the ordinary for me to have been there.

So, having written that brief story, I look back and I think through it, asking the question, "What has come of this?"

✍

Not every experience we've had in the church has led to some grand outcome today, but you'd be surprised. Sometimes a small moment in the past starts a heartbeat that still beats strong today. Sometimes an experience with the church instills a value that we find ourselves working to carry out later on. Sometimes a bad memory still scares us, years after the initial threat has passed; we often don't even realize we are reacting to something so distant. Sometimes a loving encounter serves as a model of how to love others for years to come. What has come of the events you've narrated in your story?

## Stories of Mentoring and Leadership

A third kind of story we might tell, after our stories with God and our stories with the church, is a story of how a specific person has influenced us. What people has God placed in your path? How has God used those people? Where have you been led by mentoring or the leadership of another person? And what can you learn from those examples? In this section, we'll take some time to write about our stories of mentoring and leadership.

### Draw/Jot

I like to start this activity simply by looking back at the maps and drawings I've made so far. Try looking back at the beginning of this chapter and find one of the maps or drawings you made earlier. Using a different colored pen, touch the map or drawing and, when a specific person comes to mind, write his or her name. You don't have to write more about that person right now—just the name. Spend some time doing this. Linger until you have several names. Perhaps they are pastors who led you at some point in time. Perhaps they were influential teachers, parents, or other adults who mentored you when you were young. Perhaps they were bosses or supervisors you had at a job. A supervisor at an internship, or a senior colleague. Professors who taught you. Elders in your congregation, or just in your life. Who helped you?

Or maybe it's someone who didn't exactly help you, in a direct way, but whose example has meant a lot to you. There's a person in my church right now who, although I rarely spend time with them one-on-one, I think of and look to all the time. She's more than twenty years older than me; her children are my own age. I see how she is in our congregation; I see how she is with her adult children; I see how well she listens when we're talking around the table at adult Sunday school; and I see how she takes time to give little gifts, or to bring soup to the person who's had a baby. This person, even from afar, is an example for me of how to love out loud. She never seeks to make herself important. She leads when it makes sense for her to do so, but she can also step back and be a member of the group when someone else is at the helm. She's thoughtful—much more thoughtful than I am. She remembers the little things. When she gives a gift, it has a handmade touch—a tag that she cut from fancy paper, or a little something that she's sewn, or a note she has written.

Spend some time looking at your maps and drawings, or perhaps just remembering and making a list. Once you've got a list with several people on it—perhaps some from the past and some more current—you're ready to write.

Spiritual Mentors

1. ______________________________
2. ______________________________

3. ______________________________
4. ______________________________
5. ______________________________
6. ______________________________
7. ______________________________
. ______________________________
. ______________________________
. ______________________________

### Write

Set a timer for seven minutes, or ten, or fifteen. By now you know more about your own stamina as well as how this writing time fits into the bigger picture of your day. But be realistic—almost nobody goes more than twenty minutes without losing focus. It's not a contest.

Choose one of the people on your list and hold that person in mind. When you're ready, jump in and describe that person and their action on your life. You don't need to answer all of these questions, or any of them, but if you need them, they're here to help you think:

What did they look like?
What did they wear?
What did their voice sound like?
What phrases or sayings did they repeat?
How did you meet this person?
How did they make you feel?
What did you learn from them?
What are you still learning from them?
How did you see this person interacting with others?
How did they spend time?

What activities did they avoid?
What rules or values did they espouse? Follow?
What were they like in conflict? How did they handle problems?
Where did they get energy? How did they care for themselves?
How did they challenge you? How did you respond?

If you run out of steam writing about one person, you can always switch to writing about someone else. Remember everything that you can. Keep in mind that even with someone you really appreciate, or from whom you've learned a lot, there may also be negative things to remember. That's OK; that's part of the total picture of who this person was for you, or is. When I think about my mentors in my own past, there are a lot of times that were difficult, even with folks I really appreciate and respect. Sometimes I didn't want to learn what that person was teaching me, or didn't understand something that I now see more clearly. Sometimes it's just that that person's humanness got in the way, and they were, well, *human* when I expected them to be perfect. Sometimes they were struggling with something of their own and weren't available to me the way that I wanted. That's OK; it's part of the total picture of what it was to learn from this person. When it comes to examples, the picture is always partial. We don't want to actually be another person; it's that there are things we notice in the process of witnessing another person that we wish to emulate. The clearer picture you can make of this person in your writing, the better. And don't worry about whether you're being fair to your chosen person. It's not about recording things for posterity, and nobody will see it anyway. It's about noticing what you can notice, in a way that helps you draw from your memories later on in your own actions.

✍

Read and Reflect

When your time is up, or when you feel you've run out of gas writing, or simply when you're ready to move on, here are some strategies for making use of what you have written. Of course, you can always return to one of the strategies we have used earlier in this chapter, or bring something from later in the book back to here. But for now, here are some ways you might spend time with what you have written about a mentor or leader and learn from it:

*Specific actions*

One powerful move can be to read back over your account and simply highlight specific actions this person took. You can start by going through with a colored pencil or highlighter and marking actions you mentioned. For example, when I wrote about a pastor whom I admired and learned from, who helped me discern possibilities for ministry of my own, I read back and identified these specific actions that he took that influenced me:

He *listened* to my wonderings, in a series of appointments at his office as well as in snippets of chat here and there at church dinners and events.

He *asked* me how things were going. I am not someone who easily brings up my own issues, especially with a busy person who I am mostly encountering in public spaces. So, it was really important that he actually asked me directly about my discernment process from time to time.

He *wrote* letters of recommendation and spoke on my behalf to people in connection to my candidacy.

He *preached*, not to me alone of course, but to our congregation, in ways that showed me how one man connected to the text each week and that also left space for how I might also connect to it—sometimes differently than he did. He also preached bravely, bringing up topics such as sexual orientation that I knew he sometimes feared to mention and had previously avoided. His brave example in preaching encouraged me to be brave myself in other domains, and his preaching in connection to challenging social issues helped me discern my own commitments to equity.

He *prayed* for me, in my presence and also (he told me) occasionally on his own as part of his prayer practice each morning.

When I look at this list of actions this pastor took, they really are not uncommon or unusual actions for a pastor at all: listen, ask, write, preach, pray. They're part of the job description! Yet my focus here is on how those actions affected me, and how I in turn responded to them. How did an important person in your own life influence you? What specific actions did that person take that mattered to you, whether they were intended just for you or not? Take some time to write a list of actions, or simply to freewrite with these queries in mind.

✍

*Words*

Next, read what you have written and highlight or circle any quotes you have included. That is, can you remember specific words this person has said that have stuck with you? Sometimes these are profound sayings, but sometimes they are just little turns of phrase that you might associate with that person. My former graduate school adviser, Sheridan Blau, likes to say, “Don’t try to sound smarter than you are. Just sound as dumb as you are.” I know what he means. When you try to sound smarter than you are, you end up sounding kind of stupid. If you just go with your own authentic voice, you’ll sound as smart as you are. It’s good advice. I heard him say this to classes, to audiences at workshops and presentations. I needed to hear it, every single time.

But the words don't always have to be profound. Sometimes, they just conjure the memory of that person in a vivid way. My friend Kris, from whom I have learned a lot, uses the phrase, "How 'bout it!" As in: "These are great burgers." "How 'bout it!" Or: "It's been a looooooong winter." "How 'bout it!" It's her phrase of enthusiastic agreement. I can't hear someone else say it without thinking of her.

Or there's the pastor who, knowing I was tired from stretching myself way too thin, simply said of a project I had taken on, "You know, you could quit." He said it casually; he probably doesn't remember saying it at all. But the words got through my layers of effort, pride, ambition, and performance like a piercing arrow. I could quit. I didn't, not right away, but the idea had been spoken, and there was freedom in it. I had options.

What words have your influential people said that have stuck with you? Sometimes just underlining them or jotting them down is enough. These are words you can say to yourself, even if that leader or mentor is no longer standing by. Or, they are words you can say to someone else, passing on the gift. I once heard a gifted colleague say to a student, "I have time for you." Now, I know what this colleague's calendar was like. He didn't exactly have time, extra time, for anyone or anything. But he gave that student a gift: "I have time for you." And you could see the student change as she received the gift: her shoulders lowered, her voice relaxed, and in the next few minutes (and without really taking any more time than usual), she got right to the heart of the research problem she had come in for help with. I've taken those words and now use them all the time. To the student rushing through our meeting, in the constant state of hurry college students have learned to maintain: “I have time for you.” To my seven-year-old son, tripping over his own words as he rushes to tell me about his day, or when I feel like tapping my foot as he takes forever to get his coat on: “I have time for you.” To a friend apologizing for talking about herself (why do women do this? We all need to talk about ourselves.): “I have time for you.”

Or you might write those words on a Post-it and leave them as a note to yourself. What words of mentorship would be good to recall just as you arrived at work each day? Stick them on the dashboard of your car. What words are meant for the doorframe of your apartment, to recall as you enter or leave each day? What words for the refrigerator, for the front of your day planner? Your Bible? Your cell phone?

Or maybe you’ll write one of those phrases at the top of a new page and spend another seven minutes writing. What did those words mean to you when your important person said them? What do they mean to you now?

✍

## Table of Contents / The Next Chapter

All this storying helps me to see how one's entire life can be envisioned as a story, or perhaps an anthology of stories. The experiences we have, and what we make of them, develop over time into narratives that help us to make sense of things. One more exercise helps to contextualize these stories in the bigger "story" of a life.

First, read back over one or more of the maps you made here along with its associated writing. Then, imagine this: Your life is like a book with chapters (or, if you prefer, a television series with episodes). What are the different chapters so far, and what is the title of each chapter so far?

I've tried this activity with all kinds of groups, from high school and college students, to church people at retreats, to teachers, to my own friends, and I am always amazed at how excellent these tend to be. Having written books, which means having first written and revised and cried over tables of contents for those books, I think tables of contents are really hard to write. But apparently it's just a skill I should be working on, because I always love to hear how people title their chapters.

A table of contents for a book about my years in elementary and secondary school might look something like this:

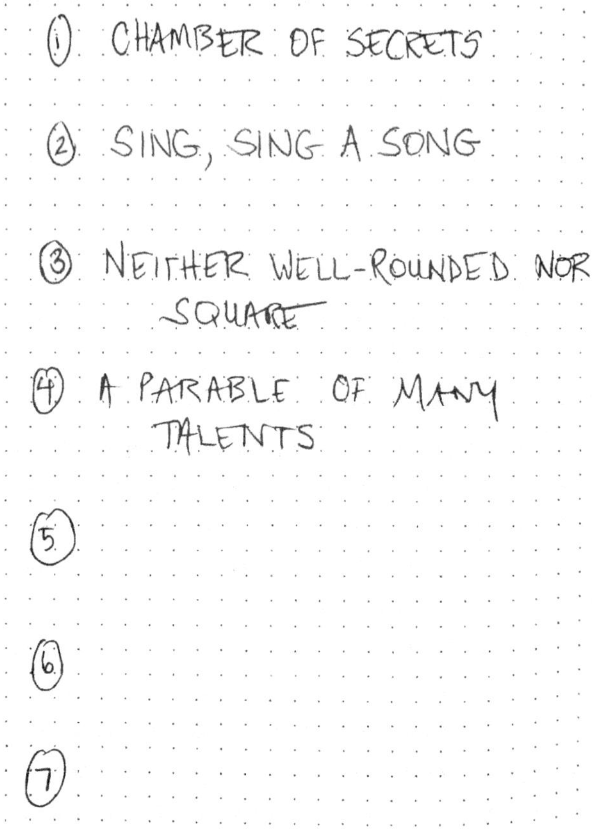
1 CHAMBER OF SECRETS
2 SING, SING A SONG
3 NEITHER WELL-ROUNDED NOR SQUARE
4 A PARABLE OF MANY TALENTS
5
6
7

1. ______________________________
2. ______________________________
3. ______________________________
4. ______________________________
5. ______________________________
6. ______________________________
7. ______________________________

. ______________________________

. ______________________________

. ______________________________

This next part is sometimes harder: What might the next few chapters be? I find that it helps to brainstorm a list of several possibilities. As I build my list (and as I look over the shoulders of people in my workshops), I see how some follow from the plot so far better than others. Some connect thematically to the rest better than others. Some are hopeful; some suggest dramatic plot twists; some are cliffhangers.

Of course none of us can know how our stories might turn out. But imagining possibilities can help us see ways to go that we might not otherwise envision. And looking back, renaming the chapters, reordering them, and revising helps us to rework our sense of what some of those earlier chapters have meant. What might have been a story of shame can become one of survival, or what seemed inevitable might now seem a bit more subject to our influence. In no way are we solo authors of our stories, but we *are* coauthors.

• • •

Taken together, this chapter has been about recalling and reflecting on stories from our lives of faith. What have you learned from writing these stories? Sometimes it's enough just to realize that we *have* stories. Our histories with God, with the church, and with other people—even people who have led or mentored us—are not simple or easy. As we age and change, so do our understandings.

# 3

# SHOWING UP

## Writing for Mindful Presence

Recently, I showed the movie *E.T.* to my children for the first time. Nine years old when it first came out, I now have seen the film many times and count it as one of my favorites. It even holds a special place in my heart because a showing in a Los Angeles theater was one of my ex-husband's and my first dates. I had an E.T. doll when I was a kid, and I've described the movie to my kids many times. I've even ridden the truly terrible E.T. ride at Universal Orlando, in which riders land on E.T.'s "home planet" and encounter happy, Ewok-like aliens, including E.T.'s "friends" who somehow do not look like E.T. at all.

Yet as I watched *E.T.* for the umpteenth time, I noticed something new. I always understood how, at the end of the movie, E.T. and Elliot are somehow telepathically connected, such that as E.T.'s health declines, so does Elliot's, and such that when E.T. accidentally gets drunk at home, Elliot burps and sways dizzily in his science classroom. But this time, I saw details I had never seen before. First, that mental/physical connection begins much sooner, on the first night E.T. enters the house. As E.T. slowly closes his eyes, he makes Elliot sleepy too. And further, with this viewing of the film, I saw more clearly than ever before the theme of the cynical older brother becoming reconnected to his siblings and to wonder and possibility. These new noticings added richly to my reading of the movie and helped me to love it even more. As I write this, I'm realizing that one reason these details, which I had experienced passively before, now seem so foregrounded is that now I am seeing the film as an adult and a parent. I see in Elliot my own son, or sometimes what I imagined about my ex-husband when he was a boy; I see in the relationships between the kids the interactions my own kids have as siblings.

Our ability to *notice* is a gift of presence. It is a gift God gives to us, that even what is seemingly familiar can yield new ideas. Yet noticing is also a gift we can in turn give. When we give this gift to another person, we say to them, "I know you; you're of interest; I am paying attention." Further, we give this gift to God by noticing, newly and with openness to new interpretations, the world and beings God has made.

This sequence of writing activities directs you to notice. The chapter invites you to show up and explore a different level of experience of your everyday being. It is natural that, in order to live, we filter out much of the information that bombards us every day. However, this can leave us disconnected from our surroundings, our experiences, and even ourselves. Writing can help us to notice, and that engages us to be more mindfully present in our days.

## NOTICING PLACES

Where are you? When asked this question, most of us will answer with the *name* of a place: "Right now I'm in my family room." "I'm at home." "I'm in State College, Pennsylvania." These statements locate us on a map (a human invention) or in a building (another manmade structure). But how much do names of places really convey about the places, and in turn what might they obscure about these places or the influence that being in a certain place may have on us?

I've lived in this house in this town for fifteen years, the longest I've lived anywhere as an adult. This kind of longevity makes a place more familiar, but on another level, it makes a place harder to see, doesn't it?

When we write with the intention of really noticing and describing the places we're in, we see them not only in more detail but also perhaps in revised detail. That is, places change, sometimes in their physical characteristics but always also in their function as contexts for our activities.

In these pages of my notebook, I just started with "I see," "I hear," "I feel," and so on, describing the room I am in right now. Sometimes I just observed some aspect of the physical space. Other times a memory popped in, and I wrote that down too.

Can you try it? Wherever you are right now, where you happen to be reading this, take a moment to notice the place that you are in. No need to overachieve: What do your senses perceive in this moment and location? If a memory pops in, jot that down too, but no need to dig for them. You're only describing right now; no need to go further. Just be in your space, and write what you notice:

Wednesday, April 22

In the family room
In my white chair
By the sunny backyard window
I see three fuzzy blankets strewn around from last night's TV watching. I hear my son making siren + explosion noises, beat boxing, narrating his Lego play, opening sentences with "Hey, mom..."
I hear parakeets chirping + squeaking, carrying on some always-ongoing conversation. Maybe, like William, they're narrating what they play and imagine.
I see their seed hulls on the carpet
I feel warmth from the sun shining in over my shoulder — welcome warmth even though it's cold outside.

I see the children's bookcases, books leaning and on their sides and many just piled in front of the bookcase, tidied up a little but not so far as actually putting them all the way away!

I see Lego toys — on a Lego table, in Lego bins, on the carpet waiting for unsuspecting feet, many dropped as if forgotten, but others in little scenes, a man with a yellow face driving some kind of space scooter away from The Incredible Hulk, or a person in a chef's hat hanging precariously from a spire atop Hogwart's, or a half-finished robot brandishing two swords.

I see carpet that has survived spit-up, ground-in Goldfish, birdseed hulls, muddy snow boots, and infrequent vacuuming.

I see the sofa we bought that barely fits, recliner left open as usual.

I hear kids yelling through the house

I see piles of books and magazines in progress

I see little rainbows on my notebook, somehow prism-ed by sun coming in the window.

I see red bricks of chimney

I see iPhone chargers

Half-alive houseplants

Reading glasses

A random sheet of bubble wrap

**What do you . . . see? hear? smell? feel?**

Every time I do this, no matter how familiar the setting, I notice something new about the space. Once you've had a chance to let your writing settle in a bit, now you can read over it. When I reread what I listed in my family room, I'm noticing how much of what I saw and heard came from my children. A Lego table is a prominent feature of our "décor," and our couch was no stylish item but instead a set of three modular recliners hooked together. This is not what I imagined my adult life would look like: In my twenties, I imagined my house in "real adulthood" being clean and light, with lots of clear surfaces, warm wooden flooring, perhaps an arrangement of fresh flowers on a coffee table. Even when I was pregnant with my oldest, my ex-husband and I swore we would not be one of those families whose entire house is packed with large, brightly colored plastic items. A baby swing right in the middle of the family room? A plastic slide indoors? Buckets of toys everywhere? No, a playroom would be enough. Kids don't need so many toys anyway.

Now in my late forties, with two children, I am living in reality. The space I'm in about half of the hours I am at home, the family room, is cluttered, a little dirty, and absolutely strewn with brightly colored plastic items. And as I realize this, I feel a hot flush of happiness. This is not what I imagined, but it is the room where everyone I love best can usually be found. All its clutter does get in my way, and every so often I anxiously scoop up a bunch of it for kids to put away elsewhere, or as fodder for a massive yard sale—but truly, the main thing I see here is evidence that my life is full of love.

Try rereading your description of a space. Anything in your writing that was new? Any surprises? What makes this space special, or what in its ordinariness have you been missing? Take some time to reflect.

✍

## NOTICING TIME

"How are you doing?"

"Busy!"

This is how virtually all conversations begin in the building where I work. They often begin this way other places I see people also: in the grocery store, in church, even by the side of the swimming pool on a summer weekday. (How busy are we really, if we have time to be at a fun pool in the middle of the week?) The feeling of being in a hurry seems like the American default now. In fact, studies show that we actually have a little more free time than we did a couple of decades ago, yet we report feeling more and more harried and pressed for time.[1,2,3] What does it mean that we feel so short on time?

Moreover, what happens to the time we do have? I've asked groups of all kinds this question: teachers, graduate students, teens, church people. I'm going to ask you too. Try making a time diary over a period of a few days. All you need is an activity and the amount of time you spent doing it.

Here's what my time log looked like on one slow work-from-home day:

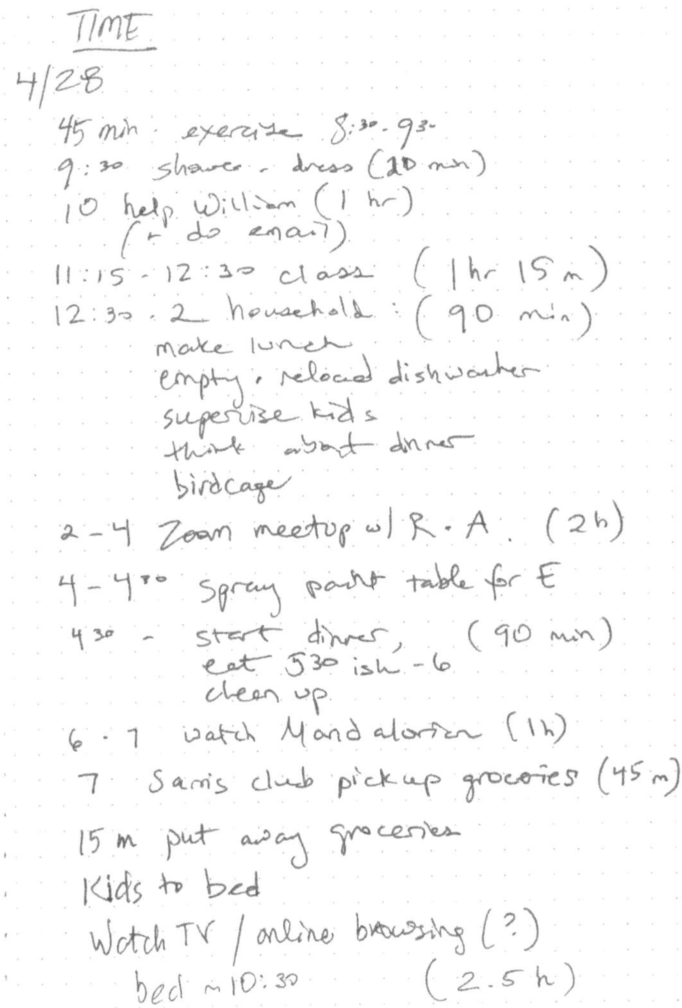

TIME

4/28

45 min exercise 8:30-9:30

9:30 shower - dress (20 min)

10 help William (1 hr)
(+ do email)

11:15 - 12:30 class (1 hr 15 m)

12:30 - 2 household: (90 min)
make lunch
empty + reload dishwasher
supervise kids
think about dinner
birdcage

2-4 Zoom meetup w/ R. A. (2 h)

4-4:30 spray paint table for E

4:30 - start dinner, (90 min)
eat 5:30 ish - 6
clean up

6 - 7 watch Mandalorian (1 h)

7 Sam's club pickup groceries (45 m)

15 m put away groceries

Kids to bed

Watch TV / online browsing (?)
bed ~10:30 (2.5 h)

Now, this exercise is not about guilt or shame. I don't have any opinion about how much time you should spend on various things. Perhaps you do, but those impressions of what should be actually may or may not be correct. So for now, try to set those aside and simply notice.

I try to do a time log every now and then: when I am starting to work toward a new goal, or when I feel overwhelmed, or when I notice myself worrying about time. Each time I do it, I am struck both by how much I am actually doing (no wonder I'm so tired!) and by how much time is spent on things that are not really worthy of it. For example, last summer I found through time logging that I was spending at least two hours each night watching TV after my kids went to bed. As my kids have gotten older and the summer nights last longer, that meant I was not getting to bed until at least 11 p.m.—and my day starts at 6 a.m.! I like that time to myself, and I also like watching TV, but that doesn't mean I have to do that every night. And, that is low-quality time (I confess I also looked at my phone while watching, often missing key parts of the story) and low-quality relaxation (I usually didn't even care what the shows were). Meanwhile, there were so many things I wanted to be doing but wasn't: tidying up before bed, writing, prayer, exercise. But mostly: sleeping. The baby step I next tried to take is to watch one show, then go up to bed, or, barring that, to read while the TV is on rather than zone out with a phone. I know it's not much, but it did make a difference. Now I'm in a place where I usually go to bed when I'm tired, while my teenage daughter stays up to watch the shows her younger brother shouldn't really see.

Where do you spend time? What do you spend it doing? How does your use of time support your values and goals, or how might it take away from them? How do devices affect our experiences of time? Take a look at your time log. Can you circle those activities that are really important for you, personally? Maybe a different color circle for things you do for others, whether for work or for significant others or someone else. Which of these activities are fun? At which of these times are you at rest? How much are you alone, and how much are you with others? I'm not arguing for any particular way of spending your time; I think that will vary depending on who you are and what your responsibilities are. But I do think you can learn a lot about what your actions show to be important to you from doing this.

✍

Jesus advised, "Where your treasure is, there your heart will be also" (Matt 6:21). I do feel like between being a parent and an employee and a spouse and a member of my communities, in the culture of the USA in the twenty-first century, that my time is a treasure.

## NOTICING BODIES

This book is about the spirit, but our spirits live in bodies and are inseparable from our bodies. What is your body doing right now? What messages does it send? How might body and spirit be better partners?

Try a body scan. There are many ways to do this, but the way I can actually remember and use regularly has to be bone-simple. So: Sit with a healthy posture wherever you happen to be. Take a couple of minutes just sitting there, enough that the grocery list and your next appointment and that bad meeting yesterday get a bit quieter, enough that your mind is a bit less squirmy and maybe your body is too. Now, start with your feet and just notice your body, part by part, until you reach the top of your head. Does anything hurt? Itch? Feel twitchy? Are you saggy, or tight, or uncomfortable? Do any parts feel good? What temperature(s) can you sense? What is touching your body now: clothing, the cool plastic of a desk chair, air from a vent nearby, hair in your eyes? Sunshine?

Now, take a few minutes (I like seven!) to jot down what you were able to notice. Some people choose to draw a basic body outline and label it, while others write out their observations in sentences and don't really use a drawing. Either way works.

I'm one of those people who has spent many years basically ignoring my body. That is, I used it and I appreciated it, engaging in sports and movement with joy, but I didn't listen to my body's messages or treat it with much respect. Injuries were to be "walked off" and foods were chosen for convenience more than health. This has changed a lot, first as I became a parent, especially through my pregnancies, in which my body became strange and unlike it had ever been, yet also suddenly impressive and amazing. It made an entire organ—a placenta—from nothing! And it made two entire people, actual human people who now walk around and ride bikes and do algebra and everything, and it made each of them using just one cell from outside of me. That's just ridiculous. I connected to my body a bit more in my early forties, when I began to have health problems. I don't take this body for granted anymore; I need it to last another forty years or more!

And I finally am starting to realize that I can learn from my body about how I am feeling. Physical sensations usually carry messages about emotions. Take a look at my own body scan writing from a summer day:

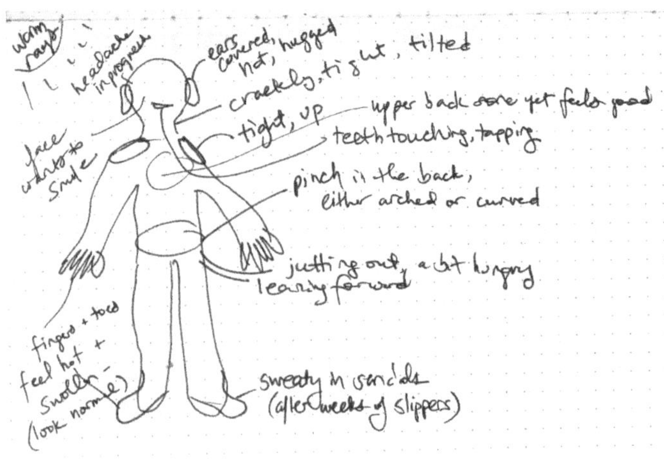

Looking over this, I have to laugh at what can be read as a list of complaints. Arthritis, and headaches, and soreness all over! And yes, I drew that body outline, and for the record, I do have two normal shoulders and typically shaped hands and feet, not quite what I've drawn here. The picture just reminds me to remember and jot what I felt when I sat still, and add what I am newly noticing as I write.

Doesn't writing do that? Many people think of writing as a way of transcribing or recording thoughts we have already produced. The truth, however, is that writing is a way of thinking. To write something is to compose as you do; even when we think we know what we mean to write, as we write we often come to understand our ideas anew or even revise our ideas altogether. So it is for me with this body scan: Based on my jottings, I am realizing how tense I really am today. Those wiggling toes, the tight shoulders, and the sore jaw are all ways my body can tell me I may be overdriving. That's my "favorite" way of coping, after all, when I am afraid of what is ahead. So, why am I feeling so tense? What am I afraid of? My body scan helps me even know to ask the question. It also gives me some hints on how I might help myself: I need some quiet prayer time, having just spent a full weekend with my children, who fill me with joy but who don't leave space for solitude. I need some exercise, as I need most every day, but maybe some stretching today, or at least some extra kindness to my shoulders. And, in turn, to my spirit.

You might try choosing one of the body parts or sensations to write about. Are there one or two that stand out? Take a few minutes and write what comes to mind: What was the sensation? What are its associations? In the example below, I wrote about my stomach.

As I sat I noticed my stomach sticking out and the littlest bit resting on my legs. I noticed that when I felt it, I immediately wanted to suck it in, adjust my pants to pull it in. I resisted the urge, but too late, I started to feel "all the feels" about it as they say. These are thoughts I wish I didn't have! Having them actually deeply offends me as a feminist! But I will voice them: WORDS like tummy, belly, pooch, mom belly, meno belly, jelly roll, flab, etc. etc. The more I write them, the more I feel ashamed that I say these to myself. Because I don't say these about other women, or even other men! How I love a good tummy on a woman. If I picture a gorgeous woman in my mind, I see a curvy one, someone with big movements, who dances with a butt that sticks out and breasts that move around. If I run through an inner catalog of women I actually know whom I find beautiful, none has a six pack, that's for sure—

they all have a yummy, pettable, woman's tummy.

Yet when I think of *myself*, my own stomach or a time when *I* was at my most beautiful, there's no belly there. I'm thin like a teenager, wearing any t-shirt and not caring how tight it goes over my front. No checking for back fat!

*Why* must I impose on myself the oppressive load of BS that society, media, men -- who? exactly -- puts on women? It's not what I like to see; I'm ashamed it's apparently what I'd like to *be*.

It's never really just a body part. Our bodies have messages to send about our feelings, past experiences, needs, and desires. Or in my case, a fair amount of feminist ranting. Not going to lie: feminist ranting is one of my better talents.

## NOTICING FEELINGS

I used to joke that when I had an emotion, I was always the last to know. I saw myself as a Spock-like character, overwhelmingly rational and driven by thought rather than "mere feelings." I was proud of this, like maybe I was above the fray of the usual human ups and downs. Maybe even worthy of space travel. Um, no. Now that we have the animated movie *Inside Out*, even a young child knows that feelings are a huge part of how we experience and engage in the world, and to try to suppress negative feelings is not only stupid but damaging.[4]

It is by feeling our feelings that we move to the other side of them, learning what we are to learn from them. Feelings are resources, information sources that tell us what we need and what we might pursue. We experience them in our thinking and in physical sensations, not only in the abstract. The key is to notice the messages and work out what they mean.

For example, I have the unfortunate habit of agreeing to do things. On its own that's not a bad thing, but I keep on agreeing and agreeing until I am overloaded. Then I resent all the people I've agreed with. Being so out of touch with my own feelings, I had no tools with which to discern what I actually wanted to do, what felt good when I did it, or what made me uncomfortable or anxious. Thus it's often my experience that it's only when a commitment has ended that I realize how much I hated it or how bad it was for me.

We've already done some writing that can give us insight into our emotions, particularly in the body scan we conducted in the previous section. Look there again—are there physical signs listed there that connect to emotions? For example, a migraine and an aching jaw usually can tell me I am worrying, even when I am not really aware of it. My eyes get sort of squinty, my forehead furrowed, when I am too tired. When I'm going back and forth between fridge and pantry, but nothing sounds good to eat, I am actually overwhelmed, and it would be best to just sit down and close my eyes for a few minutes. Look back at your own body scan—what clues to emotions are there?

It turns out that you need vivid vocabulary for writing about emotions just as you do for any other topic. To write about writing, you need terms like "revise," "draft," and so on; to write about gymnastics, you need words like "handspring," "extension," "layout," "amplitude," or "dismount." To write about feelings, you're going to need more items in your toolkit than happy, sad, mad, and glad. Psychologist Robert Plutchik developed a frequently adapted "emotions wheel" of human feelings in relation to one another; you can see a variety of representations of it with a simple web search.[5] Many creative writers have used it to develop rich characters, and I find it useful in getting precise about emotions in any kind of writing.[6]

Try this: Think about a situation in your life on which you'd appreciate some insight. You can describe the situation in the space below. Then, gather (from your own vocabulary or from a list) specific emotion terms that fit your feelings within this situation. Many terms will apply; try to identify them all. Don't worry if some of your choices seem to conflict with one another; feelings don't necessarily fit into a tidy package.

Describe a situation on which you'd like some insight:

List emotion words associated with the situation:

In my own example, I focused my own writing on uncertainty about an upcoming sabbatical from my university. I needed to make a chain of decisions, and I was having trouble sorting through all the factors. Here's what I wrote:

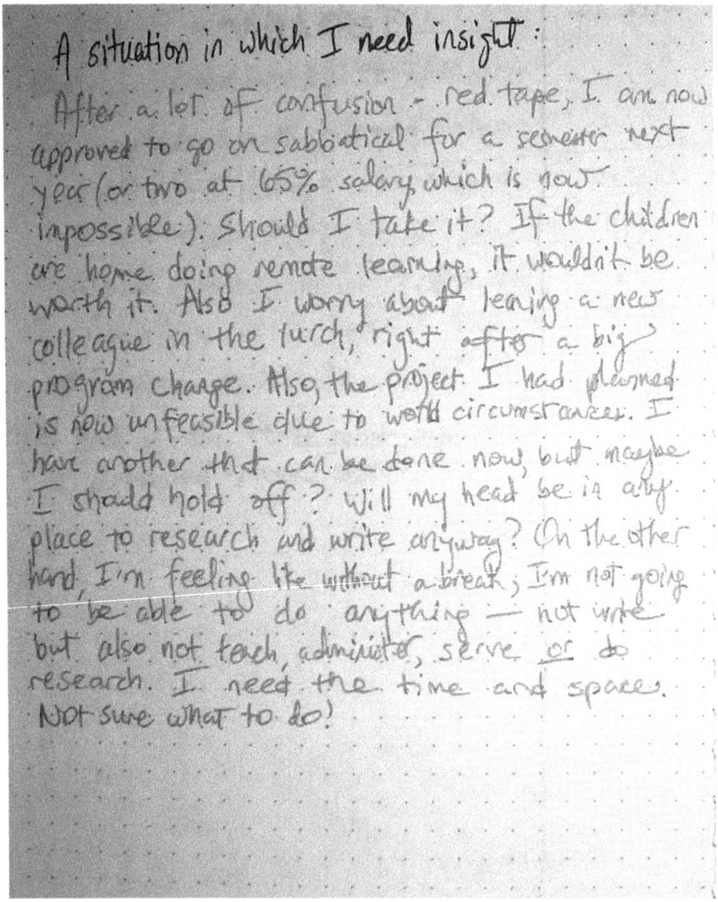
A situation in which I need insight:

After a lot of confusion + red tape, I am now approved to go on sabbatical for a semester next year (or two at 65% salary, which is now impossible). Should I take it? If the children are home doing remote learning, it wouldn't be worth it. Also I worry about leaving a new colleague in the lurch, right after a big program change. Also, the project I had planned is now unfeasible due to world circumstances. I have another that can be done now, but maybe I should hold off? Will my head be in any place to research and write anyway? On the other hand, I'm feeling like without a break, I'm not going to be able to do anything — not write but also not teach, administer, serve or do research. I need the time and space. Not sure what to do!

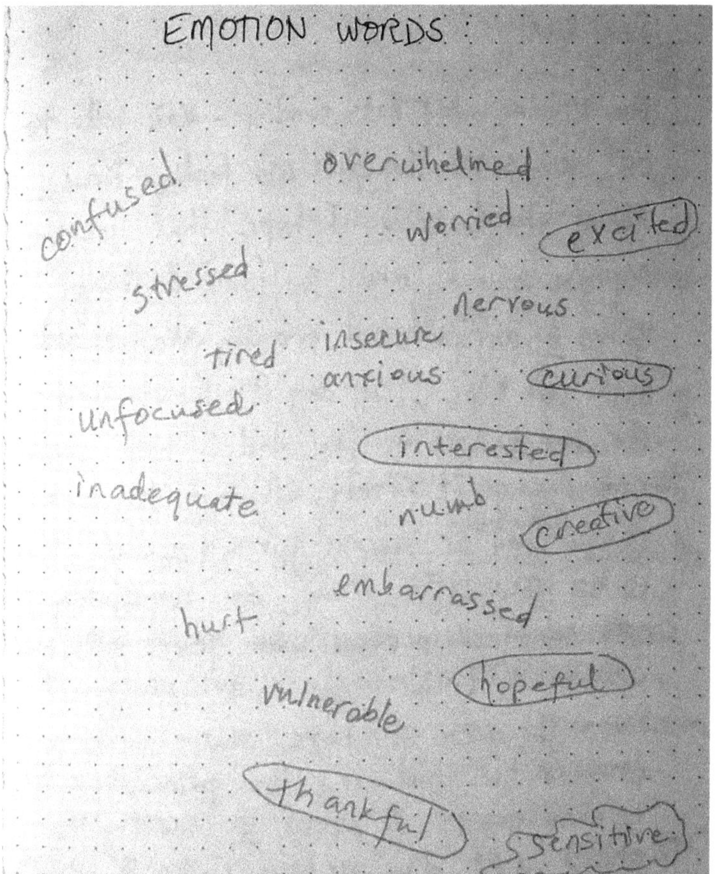
EMOTION WORDS
confused
overwhelmed
worried
excited
stressed
nervous
tired
insecure
anxious
curious
unfocused
interested
inadequate
numb
creative
embarrassed
hurt
hopeful
vulnerable
thankful
sensitive

These decisions around the sabbatical were really fraught for me, as you can tell. I feel so lucky to even have a job where such an opportunity exists; however, I also feel a lot of (mostly self-imposed) pressure to make excellent use of it—and that's where I run into trouble. What is the best way to use this gift? The best time? What are factors (few of which I control) that make this a good or bad time to take it?

Once you've got your own list, here are some questions you can use to go deeper:

- What category(ies) dominates your list?
- Are some feelings much stronger than others? Which ones?
- What surprises did you find in your list of feelings, if any?
- Are there factors outside of the actual situation that might be influencing your feelings about it?
    - What accounts for any outside factors, surprises, strong feelings, and/or dominating categories?
    - If you were to make a decision or act on this situation based on emotions information alone, what decision or action would you take?

As I look back over my description and then the words I drew from the emotions wheel, I can see that I have many more negative-tinted words than positive ones. In fact, I circled all of the positive words (and put a wavy line around one I found ambiguous) to check whether my impression was correct. Now, the emotion wheel itself has many more negative emotions than positive in the first place—a result of the bias toward negativity that we carry from earlier days in human evolution, in which negative emotions were signals that conveyed likely threats of danger and thus were especially important to pay attention to. Writing can help us attend to our emotions and their messages for us. It helps us find out what we feel in the first place, and it helps us learn from and move through the feelings. What do these words help you to notice, and perhaps name, about your emotions regarding a topic?

✍

## NOTICING OTHERS

When we mindfully attend to our own experience, we quickly see others in a new light as well. I remember that, when my first child was born, I kept having this feeling that everyone had previously been a baby. It changed everything. I was once a baby, and my mom, with whom my relationship has had some difficult parts, felt about me the way I feel about this child, no matter how complicated it got later on. And *she* was also a baby, loved and tiny and held in just the same way, no matter how things changed after that. That person at work who just has to be cantankerous about every idea ever brought up at a meeting? Yep, someone's baby. A loved one, in an argument? Baby. Stranger having a tantrum at the checkout counter? Baby.

Somehow, imagining all people as former babies made me nicer to them in my head. While on the outside I might not have done anything different, on the inside my whole tone of voice changed. I could say silently, "You're screwing up. But you're a loved child of God." It made me more compassionate, or even more forgiving. Or it helped me get curious instead of judgmental: I could think, "Wow, I wonder what happened in your life that made you feel that way," or "Who spoke to you the way you are speaking so harshly now?" We were all babies once, lovable and helpless and squishy and filled with the hopes of everyone who loved us. It was obvious back when we were newborns that we were God's children; as we get older, though, this can sometimes be harder and harder to see. At least if you're grumpy and misanthropic like I often am.

A writing task that helps me adjust how I am thinking about someone else is the "unsent letter."[7] Really, the main thing keeping me from seeing all people as the babies of God I know them to be is . . . my relationships with those people. That grumpy colleague? She has power over me, and that makes me anxious. My kids? I fear every step will indelibly mark their futures, and that makes me crazy. Writing an unsent letter is a way of stepping outside a relationship to consider someone anew. Try this:

Draft a letter to someone with whom you've had trouble (either trouble between you or simply trouble in your head). You won't be sending the letter, so you can let go of worrying about explaining why you are writing, whether they would understand, or how it would be interpreted by them or anyone else in your lives. Just center your mind on this person, and write directly to them.

You might consider writing in your letter about:

- Your hopes for them
- Your regrets about them
- Your questions about them
- What you see in them that others may not see
- What you wish they knew about you
- What you wish they knew about someone else
- . . . Or anything else that comes to mind when you think of this person

Dear Kat,

I'm writing – but not sending – this letter to tell you some thoughts and feelings I'm having about you. I hope that you are enjoying being a mom. I found the baby years so difficult, but overall, with time and with two kids, I can say it's the very best role I've had in my life. And I hope you can engage it freely, without too much comparison or second-guessing yourself. There is no one right way, so hopefully you can not feel anxious when you're not sure what's right. Nobody is, not really. I know I seem to have such strong convictions, but it's the principles or [illegible] I feel so certain

✍

I always find that these letters make me more honest. If I go ahead and say in the letter what I have chosen not to say aloud, I can say it clearly and freely. I have permission. In fact, in letters like these, I often defuse the issues for myself just by naming them. This activity helps writers notice, honor, and gain insight into another person. How might mindfully noticing another person change our relationship to that person?

## NOTICING GOD

"God is like the wind; you can't see it but you see the branches swaying."

Not going to lie, I always hated this explanation of why God doesn't appear more clearly to us. Especially when I was a teenager, raised without faith but becoming more and more hopeful that God did indeed exist, I really wanted to *know* God was there. If you want people to believe in you, I would ask the God-who-may-or-may-not-exist, why don't you make it more obvious that you are real? As time has passed, I don't feel I need to see God with my eyes in order to have faith, but as a Christian, I do find it ironic: My whole tradition is based on God becoming incarnate, appearing on Earth in a physical body. But we have no images of Jesus that survived from that time; nobody seems to have made a statue in his image or done a quick sketch and stuffed it into a jar in some cave for us to discover. Wouldn't it have been easier (and more persuasive!) to incarnate yourself in a time and place that had things like sound recorders and cameras?

Yet I know I am not alone in persisting in the belief, or at least the desire to believe, that God is here. Sometimes I'm convinced by the actions of another person who made me feel loved in the unreasonable, unconditional, "even-though" way that I am told God loves me. Sometimes it is in a beautiful moment, or beautiful sound, or beautiful vision, that I just can't accept is the result of random combinations of physical phenomena. Sometimes it's in my own body, a sense of connectedness to something beyond, or to an aspect of myself that can't possibly have come from me alone.

At the beginning of my faith journey, this would have seemed way too woo-woo for me. Sometimes I still see it that way. And I'm aware also that some faith traditions have a currently incarnated God to look at, or find the problem unimportant. And I know that many people who are seeking to engage in spiritual writing and thus are using this book have no religious tradition at all; you can be agnostic or an atheist or just an uncommitted spiritual person and still find these ways of writing meaningful. So, how might writing help us notice God?

My answer, and our writing prompt, is simple: Where do you notice things that strike you as evidence of God? Suggestive of God? Representative of God?

✍

Or, replace God with "the Divine?"

Or, with "a spiritual level of consciousness?"

Or, "the unexplainable?"

I find it matters less what you call it and more what you notice. I know lots of ways of doing this writing:

- One friend's family talks about it each night at the table: "Where did you encounter God today?" They note these sightings in a family notebook.
- I sometimes write about "when could you have called on God today?" (I tend to miss these opportunities, because I get caught up in whatever my day-to-day activities are, but when I return to them at the end of the day, not only do I see moments that I could have called on God, but I also see moments where God must have been there whether I called or not.)
- Another way is to observe scenes where God is known to have shown up in the past: churches, mountaintops, sacred art, or other sites and artifacts with significance in your religious tradition. Notice what you notice: "What stands out at this worship service? When you read these words of Scripture? When you view this icon, this statue, this symbol?"

• • •

Remember in *Pee-wee's Big Adventure*, when Pee-wee's prized red bike is stolen? Once it's gone, Pee-wee sees bikes all around him. Bikes in front of him, behind him, everywhere. The more often I write about where I notice God, the more I notice God.

# 4

# EVERYDAY DISCERNMENT

What is my life's work? What is my purpose, in general or in a specific area, like career or family? Which of these pathways should I take? How do I make this decision when none of the options seems right? And for the person of faith: What does God want from my life? And what does God call me to do *today*?

These questions all center on the theme of discernment—that is, considering purposes, exploring possibilities, and making decisions with God's help, when it's not readily clear how to interpret or act on a situation.

The metaphor of sight—and its cousin, insight—has long been used to understand what discernment means. Paul explains in 1 Corinthians 13:12, "For now we see in a mirror, dimly, but then we will see face to face. Now I know only in part; then I will know fully, even as I have been fully known." Paul compares our knowledge of God and possibly everything to the process of coming to see more clearly: first, in a dim mirror or perhaps a dirty pane of glass (or, as Eugene Peterson has imagined it, "squinting in a fog, peering through a mist" [MSG]). With the passage of time and a loving, faithful outlook, we will come to see God as well as one sees a person face-to-face, and our understanding of God will be akin to God's understanding of us. I imagine this clarity of insight to mean seeing in a way that is fully attentive to context; fully aware of all possibilities, influences, and implications; imaginative and expansive; generous in interpretation; and loving in characterization.

Writing, in and of itself, is preprogrammed to provoke a new way of seeing: It's even in our process terms like *revise*. Literally, it means "see again." While it's not necessary to get technical about this for it to work, most scholars who have considered the effect of writing on insight or decision-making describe it something like this: When you write something, you also as a matter of necessity are considering its meaning, how to frame it, what it connects to, and its implications. You use this ongoing, mostly unconscious analysis just to form the sentences and choose the words within them. For example, if, remembering and writing about a storm, I recall that I was afraid, I might call the storm "terrible"; if I remember feeling more amazed by a powerful display of lightning, maybe I'll write that it was "huge" or "impressive" or "dramatic." Then, as a matter of course while writing, we are also always reading back. As you think what to write next, you read back a few words or even sentences so that the next words and sentences will make sense from there. Finally, once we have written something, we have externalized it, and it is now more available to analyze and either act on or perhaps revise. Writing involves turning thoughts and experiences into thinner streams than the wide waterfall or ocean current that begins in our minds; when laid out on paper, single strands of thought and feeling can be followed, rearranged, and perhaps reweaved into new patterns. This quality of writing is one significant part of the mechanisms that makes it therapeutic, useful for reflection and even transformation.[1,2]

The writing practices that follow are all aimed at helping us know more about what is going on with ourselves and with situations or choices that we face. None of us is in full control when it comes to living a life. Add the divine into the mix, and it can be absolutely paralyzing to make decisions that take us the ways we *want* to go, feel we *should* go, or are *called* to go.

## DECISION MAP

Remember in chapter 2 when we mapped stories? Maps work well here also—by tracing the pathways of choice and chance that we have followed to reach a present point, sometimes we can gain insight on turns to take into the future.

With a current or upcoming decision point in mind, think about the pathway that has led you to this point. Can you draw it in the form of a road map? Some roads you have traveled may have landmarks along them. And sometimes you know what you missed along other ways you did not choose. There may also be forks in the road where one way was taken but the other fades off into the unknown.

Sometimes these maps can help us notice patterns in how we have been traveling. For example, one writer showed his map to the group, interpreting each of his choices along the way as taking "the safe road." Maybe it was or maybe it wasn't, but in his assessment we could hear that he was also disappointed in this. I saw a young woman, newly single after an engagement had ended, notice that most of her turning points weren't exactly decision points at all; they were points where she could have made a decision but, by not making one, ended up following her boyfriend's preference until the opportunity to explore her own had passed.

Sometimes when I have done this exercise, my insight has been not so much rethinking or regretting past decisions, but instead feeling gratitude for them. Choices I may have regretted at one time, I now can see that had I not made them, I might have missed out on things that did happen that I'd never want to lose. And gratitude can be a decision too, can't it?

Or, "walking" the roads on the map can show me strategies I didn't know I had in my toolkit, but now with insight could use more intentionally. Like when I looked at one map and thought, whoa, the better choices were the times I let more time pass before choosing. I really hadn't known that. I tend to be so uncomfortable with undecided things that I hurry up and intensely decide. When circumstances prevented me from jumping the gun like that, I ended up happier with my choice later on. Seeing that, I now try hard to slow myself down. Most big choices can wait a month, or a couple of weeks, or a couple of days . . . and almost every decision can stand to be slept on for one night. This is the life-course equivalent of leaving an item in my online shopping cart for a day or two, knowing that if I forget it's there, I must not really have needed it.

## DISCERNMENT TIMELINE

Here's another way of mapping. Think about the topic you're trying to better understand or to make decisions about. There's the current decision, and then there's a longer-term theme or topic of which this moment or decision is one example. I spent a period considering whether I might enter ordained ministry in my denomination (theme: vocation and work); I've considered whether to buy this house, or that vacation, or this activity for my kids, or an unnecessary new TV (theme: money); I've had to decide on major moves such as going back to school or moving across the country (theme: location); I took years figuring out whether I might improve my marriage or decide to divorce (theme: family and identity).

What's your topic? In other words, what core theme runs through the decisions you are facing now? People I've worked with in classes and retreats have identified issues like relationship, career, money, education, drinking/drugs/substances, family, and more. Once you've got your topic or theme that underlies your discernment, you can write it in the center top of a page, like this, with an additional horizontal line halfway down, like this:

**Theme:** ____________________

Then, think of that top line as a timeline. Along it, name some of the important events or decisions of your past in relation to that theme. For example, for teaching (a career in which I've had several different positions and situations), I've been considering several changes in what and when I teach as well as the timing of a long-anticipated sabbatical. Yet it's hard to know quite what is best. Am I thinking through a veil of exhaustion, and I might feel differently after some time away? I listed some key events in my own history that I remembered as relevant decision points or relevant to decision points. Mine included some of the times I really realized I enjoyed teaching enough to do it as a career, some strong experiences with colleagues (positive and negative), some turning points along my way as a teacher for the past twenty-three years, some especially memorable classes, and so on. These I laid out in something as close to chronological order as I could. Keep in mind, it's not terribly important that they be in the right order. You're making the timeline in order to recall the items on it, and then we'll use it further from there once the memories are there.

Once the timeline is fleshed out, the next step is to read it over as a whole unit and notice what you can from there. These ideas can be written in the remaining space below your timeline. When I do this, I usually start by noticing my overall impressions of points on the timeline: Was this a good time, or a bad one? That's overly reductive, but it helps me to also notice and write the associations that I have with that time. In one teaching job, I had my so-called "dream job," but I also had panic attacks on the way to work. One of my events stands out because it shows a beloved mentor, whose influence on me was/is so great that I still find myself saying words he would say and wanting to call him to ask his advice even though I am now a veteran professor and he is well past the typical age of retirement. This bottom half of the page is a place to put all those feelings and associations that bubble up as I constructed my timeline and as I further review it now. Can you try it with your own timeline? As you think of the events on it, what feelings arise—Pride? Shame? Worry? Regret? Gratitude? What do good events have in common? What do bad events have in common? Work your way down the line, noting what comes up. Here's my example:

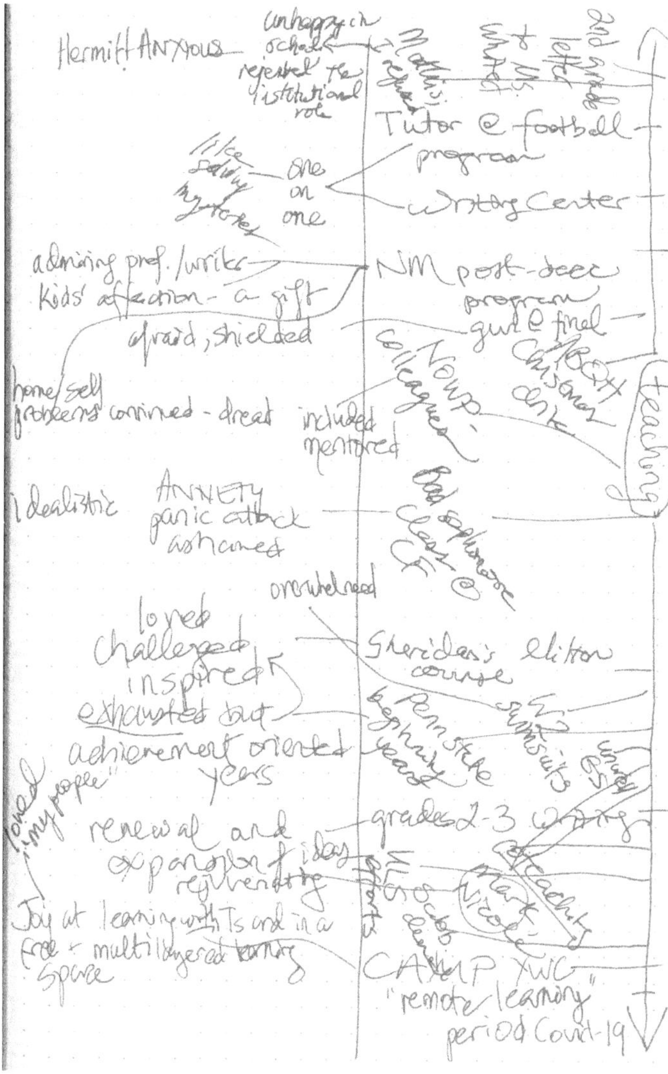


Top of image

I'm ready to reflect and write about what I might take from it. I'm just going to the next page in my notebook; you can do it below. Take a few minutes to quickwrite about what this exercise could be showing you. If you're not sure, you can write "I'm not sure, but *maybe* . . ." and see where the sentence takes you. Does it reveal anything that is worth taking into consideration in your decision-making now?

One thing this helps me to see is how much anxiety threads through my teaching history. Sometimes I've faced it, sometimes run from it. Always a consideration, but not easy to tell how to respond. My baseline is anxious — but sometimes it's a <u>real</u> message that something I'm planning or doing is not a fit. I haven't always been a good listener to myself.

I also notice how good things are when the right kind of person/people are around. Not in HS, not teaching W2 or tutoring FB. But at other times WP people, YWC, Colleen, Deana, my years with Sheridan — these are times of growth or even blossoming like a new butterfly with love + great questions and camaraderie all around as I work hard and learn. This is so different from other times in my teaching life in which I've been alone, or at least <u>felt</u> alone even though people (even good people!) may have been nearby if I'd looked. So from this I

*Example continued from previous page:*

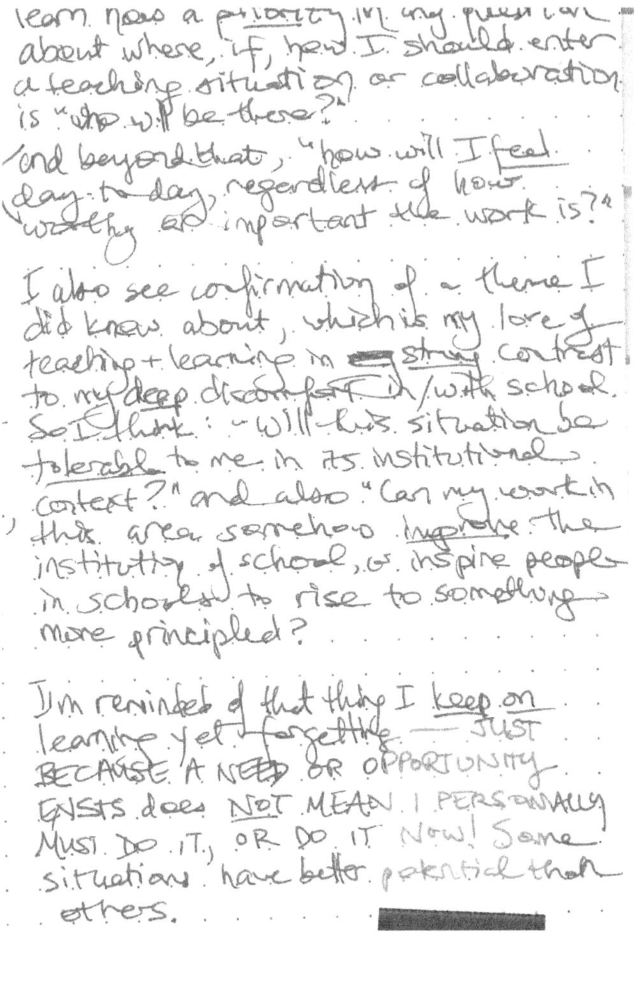

learn now a priority in my questions about where, if, how I should enter a teaching situation or collaboration is "who will be there?"

and beyond that, "how will I feel day to day, regardless of how worthy or important the work is?"

I also see confirmation of a theme I did know about, which is my love of teaching + learning in strong contrast to my deep discomfort in/with school. So I think: "Will this situation be tolerable to me in its institutional context?" and also "Can my work in this area somehow improve the institution of school, or inspire people in schools to rise to something more principled?

I'm reminded of that thing I keep on learning yet forgetting — JUST BECAUSE A NEED OR OPPORTUNITY EXISTS does NOT MEAN I PERSONALLY MUST DO IT, OR DO IT NOW! Some situations have better potential than others.

## SCENARIOS MENU

I frequently have a student sitting across from me who is struggling to decide something. Which research topic should I pursue? This decision influences how they spend their time for the next two years and position you in a tough job market after graduation. Or, which job should I apply for, or take? It often comes down to two or three dramatically contrasting offers, in different parts of the country and with different foci, or more commonly, between one bird-in-the-hand offer and a hoped-for possibility of something better coming down the road. What to do? Ironically, the more choices we have, the more difficult our decision-making becomes and the more stress we experience.[3] Further, it turns out that we are not that good at thinking through what the outcomes of decisions will be, so when we finally do decide, we often do so based on bad information. How to discern among any set of choices with such a spotty basis for the choice? What's more, the more we're aware of our own propensity for making bad choices, the more fearful of the decision points we may become. This is how we can end up on the sofa gobbling pretzels in our pajamas watching Netflix when something really important is looming. Please don't tell me I'm the only one.

When my students reach these decision points and get stuck, I assign "the scenarios menu." It is an exercise in imagination that helps add needed information in situations like this. Prepare a "menu" of choices, treating each option in a paragraph or two each. Make the descriptions of each option as thick as you can: If it's a research proposal, I ask them to point to key sources and study design. If it's a move, do the cost-of-living calculations and research the location so that you know what you're talking about. If it's adding on a commitment or taking one away, consider the activity itself, but also consider outcomes ranging from money, to time, to your body, to relationships. What will you *not* do because you're doing this? And consider that there are rarely just two options; most life decisions are not yes/no choices. There are in-betweens—in fact, it's failure to consider the in-betweens that usually gets me into trouble!

My students invariably find that one or two menu options are way easier to write than the others. This is usually because that idea or those ideas are better than the rest. Or, just as informative to note, those ideas are more fun to think about than the other ideas. Sometimes one option is simpler in some important way that makes it more practical. That's a clue, isn't it? If you can't get interested in two paragraphs about this project idea, how will you engage it for two years? Having written the menu of scenarios gives the student a handle on what it would actually be like to spend time working on that thing, how interested they actually are in it, or whether they were only considering it because they thought it would please someone else. Similarly, for me when I'm discerning whether to add a project to my already heaping plate, writing out the various possible scenarios helps me amplify and notice how I actually feel about the activity. That project that I "should" join because it's a good opportunity, or because *someone* really should do it? Writing out and inhabiting what it might be like to actually do that work often shows me that I would be miserable doing it. Some things we just want done, not necessarily that we want to or need to do them ourselves. When that insight comes, I can genuinely and comfortably hand the project off for someone else. When I find myself excited by the scenario, then I can set myself to the task of figuring out what doing it will take. Either way, I am acting with my eyes open to the situation itself and to my own stake in it and needs. How I wish all of my life's decisions had been made with such clarity.

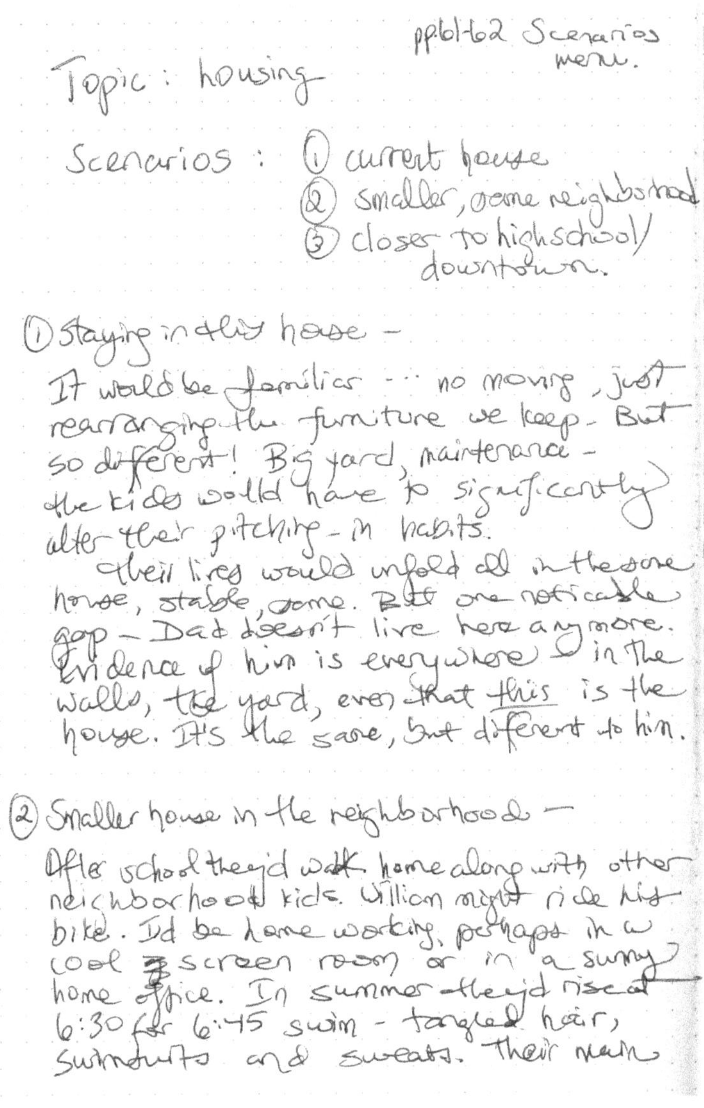

pp.61-62 Scenarios menu.

Topic: housing

Scenarios: (1) current house
(2) smaller, same neighborhood
(3) closer to highschool/downtown.

(1) Staying in this house —
It would be familiar ... no moving, just rearranging the furniture we keep. But so different! Big yard, maintenance — the kids would have to significantly alter their pitching-in habits.
Their lives would unfold all in the same house, stable, same. But one noticeable gap — Dad doesn't live here anymore. Evidence of him is everywhere — in the walls, the yard, even that <u>this</u> is the house. It's the same, but different to him.

(2) Smaller house in the neighborhood —
After school they'd walk home along with other neighborhood kids. William might ride his bike. I'd be home working, perhaps in a cool screen room or in a sunny home office. In summer they'd rise at 6:30 for 6:45 swim — tangled hair, swimsuits and sweats. Their main

hangout just a quick trip away. I may or may not go – no need to drive. The house would be clean, uncluttered, patchwork, homey. It would be new for a new start, but in the same familiar location with friends.

③ House downtown/closer to the HS –
In high school, 1 year – 5 years from now, it might be just like #2 for the kids and their worlds. (But swim for Welch? *What*?) At first, I'd ~~be~~ driving to every morning and afternoon *and* picking E~~[illegible]~~ up in the afternoons. *Ouch*. ~~But~~ we could walk downtown, etc. or even switch kids to EP/MNMS. House would be more valuable down the road, but also older with more things to fix. Smaller + less space.

It's obvious which one I want!!

✍

## WHAT'S THE WORST THAT COULD HAPPEN?

The last of these discernment strategies is a variation on envisioning scenarios. In this case, it's about looking hard at fear head-on. So much of our decision-making—or our avoidance—is actually based on fear. Fear of embarrassment, of failing, of not being loved, of losing someone's respect—whatever it is that sends you hiding, these feelings are real and come from truth, but they also tend to become exaggerated in our minds and hearts, clouding our vision. For this reason, I like to ask, "What's the worst that could happen?"

We had to decide whether to accelerate our then-five-year-old son directly from kindergarten to second grade, where he would be six among children who were seven and eight. Academically, it was definitely appropriate, but we struggled with what was right for him socially. Would he be tiny and made fun of? Would his youth, combined with his weird humor and his shoulder-length wildman hairdo, make it hard for him to have friends? Would he miss his old friends from kindergarten? Would there be gaps in his knowledge from things he would miss in first grade? What about sports—would it matter that he would someday play school sports with older (and bigger) boys, or that on age-group teams he would never be with his classmates? Would he be tall and athletic like his father, or short and scrawny like me, and would that matter? Heck, would he even care about sports? We worried and worried.

Finally the question came to me: *What's the worst that could happen?* I spent some time writing, talking with anyone who would listen, and writing some more. I came to see that the worst that could happen might be that my son would be unhappy. Other children might not accept him, or they could even be mean to him. In short, the worst that could happen was that we could advance him and then regret it. And my son would be friendless and sad, and possibly come to dread going to school, or become a target of some kind. I cried as I wrote all of this . . . and I remembered times I had not fit in, times I had wanted a friend, and times I had not enjoyed school.

In your own discernment, what's the worst that could happen? Let the fear play out in your mind. If you did take an action you are contemplating, would you lose your job? End up broke? Experience physical harm, or harm someone else? Disappoint someone you love? Fall short of your own expectations for yourself? Look stupid? Waste some time? Imagine the worst that could happen. In writing, describe that "worst" as well as you can. What would happen? How would you feel?

✍

Spend some time reading and contemplating what you write. Try to let yourself feel the feelings and see the images. Then, ask yourself these two tough questions:

- If this happened, how would you respond? Would you be OK?
- How likely is this really to happen?

In the case of our son, that first question stumped us for a while. How would we help a little boy without friends? How would we even know what scars his little soul was forming, much less what to do about them? But then, in a meeting with the school principal, the principal said something we truly had not thought of: if it didn't go well, we'd move him back. The decision was not permanent; at any time we could put him back with his old friends in the previous grade, switch him to a different class, change him to one of the other great schools nearby to have a kind of "gap year" before rejoining his original class, or creatively mix his day between the two grades, as had been arranged for our other child a few years before. Suddenly we felt more open to the experiment of advancing him. The stakes were no lower—it was still our son, whose development we wanted to nurture. Yet we felt much more agency in the situation. If an unwanted outcome came up, we had an idea how we could respond, and we knew we (and he) could live with the consequences of the choice.

As for the second question, once we honestly asked, "How likely is this worst-case scenario?" we had to admit it wasn't very likely. Our frightened visions of kids bullying and of a sad little boy left out were real things that do happen, but they weren't all that real in this case. For one thing, we actually knew a lot of the kids in the older group already, for many were siblings of our other child's friends. Second, and probably most important, we knew our son. He is ridiculously charming. He's funny, he doesn't mind being different, and he's shown that he can roll with change. We saw how our fears were somewhat likely for a generic kid in a situation like this, but not near as likely for *our* kid in *this* situation. This too, helped us move forward.

You'll find discernment in your responses to these questions: If this happened, how would you respond? Would you be OK? How likely is this really to happen? Spend some time writing about each one. Feel any clearer?

## PERSPECTIVE SHIFT

There's a cartoon I have seen again and again online in which one man is stranded on a tiny desert island, and another man is approaching on a tiny boat. The man on the island exclaims, "A boat!" The man on the boat exclaims, "Land!"

Our perception of so many things depends on perspective. Visit a place that intimidated you in childhood—say, the principal's office—and to an adult, it looks much smaller now. A medium-sized dog is like a horse to a toddler, the two standing eye to eye. Moments that seem insignificant when you're in them end up important when recalled in the wider context of a life story. And what looks easy to you might be extremely difficult for someone else.

Perspective-taking is something most adults have gotten pretty good it; it's a key component of our ability to empathize and have meaningful relationships with others. However, sometimes when it comes to our own lives, we get stuck. This possibility for writing to discern speaks to that problem; it involves deliberately writing from multiple perspectives and noticing what comes out in the differences.

I think I'm a pretty nice person. I have friends! And manners! And have no full-on enemies that I know of! But when it comes to myself, I can be mean. Mean like a power-hungry queen bee in a middle school cafeteria. Whatever empathy, grace, or generosity I show to others, I figure I shouldn't need it. I should just be better. Case in point: I decided to begin attending seminary part time. Some courses would be online, and others would be held at the seminary almost three hours from home, over country roads that may or may not be plowed. It would cost money. I was also a more-than-full-time professor at a university where the standard for producing published research is high and where women with families have often struggled to succeed, if they even chose such a career path at all. Oh yeah, I also had two kids in elementary school at that time, kids who expected things like food to eat, clothes to wear that didn't smell too bad, and rides to their never-ending stream of activities all over town. Did I mention I also had health issues causing constant fatigue at that time? Oh yeah, and a book contract, with a deadline that was starting to get pretty scary as it approached.

Obviously, it was the perfect time to start a new degree program in a new field, something completely outside of my current expertise, and in an online class format I had never experienced from the student side. And did I mention the seminary was newly configured, with its distance program mostly new, and that I did not have an academic adviser there for a whole set of reasons? Oh yes, and also the topic of my first course: biblical Greek. Why not learn a new language—heck, why not a new alphabet?—online, and right now?

Guess how that went. It turns out that it actually is possible to learn Biblical Greek in an online course, at least enough of it to find your way around various translations and points of argument among scholars surrounding this word or that one. People do it, especially with an excellent teacher, as the stream of graduates now emerging from that program makes clear. I was not one of those people. I found myself trying to do Greek poolside at the YMCA while my kids swam, over my shoulder in the kitchen while packing lunches, and from my office during certain boring webinars (ssshhhh). But mostly, truly, I found myself doing Greek the night before anything was due, in a big hurry. Usually way past my bedtime. Let's just say it was a suboptimal learning environment. I earned a C in the course, and I am pretty sure some of that was just points for showing up. Did I mention I have a PhD in education and spend my time studying, learning, and teaching? Not a good look.

Here are some of the things my head said to me during and after that experience: You idiot. Why don't you work harder? Why can't you do this? Get organized. You're such a slacker. You're wasting this opportunity. If you fail at the beginning, what do you think will come after? Try harder. Why aren't you working on Greek right now? You're going to be embarrassed. You should be ashamed. How stupid.

This, to say the least, was not a fun head to hang out in. What's more, I was so frozen in these thoughts that they played and replayed in a loop, blocking out any space I might have made to reflect on my situation and possibly make a change. Writing from different perspectives can help.

Think of a situation you are struggling with or a decision you are worrying about. Get yourself quiet and notice what your mind has to say about it; if you have written about it elsewhere in this book, you could go back and reread that. Go ahead; take a few minutes.

Now, choose another person, someone in your life whom you respect. Someone who loves you, or someone you trust. Here are some ideas:

- Your best friend
- A parent
- A mentor
- God
- Your doctor
- Your child

What would that person have to say? Think for a moment on who they are. What are their priorities, their values? What do they want for you? Now, spend some time writing in the voice of that person. What would they say to you if they heard what your head has been saying? If they knew all that you were feeling in your situation?

✍

✍

The truth about discernment is that we never actually *know* just what to do, do we? We are called, we feel led, we deduce, we have hunches, we are invited. Writing about it just makes it easier to hear those invitations.

# 5

# WRITING IN DEVOTION AND PRAYER

In some ways, writing for prayer will be the mode of spiritual writing that readers of this book find most familiar. Prayer and meditation are probably one of the first things that come to mind when we try to think of spiritual practices, right? On the other hand, my research on the writing lives of pastors showed that writing for prayer is probably not that familiar in terms of actually having much experience doing it. When the pastors I spoke to thought of writing for prayer, they tended to envision one kind of writing only: first-person journaling that resembles a diary. What's more, most reported that this was a practice they "should" be doing, but didn't, and this report was usually accompanied by guilt and shame.

The truth about writing and prayer is that while a diary-like journal in which we tell God about our activities can be one valuable way to pray, there are others. In this chapter, we'll play with strategies using writing for prayer that are varied, doable, and meaningful. None of these strategies on its own would compose an entire life of prayer. However, each adds a way of making prayer more accessible, more productive, and/or more regular.

A note about prayer from my perspective: Of course different spiritual traditions have different ideas about prayer. As a younger person, if you'd asked me what prayer was, I might have said "talking to God." As time has passed, I came to revise that to "communication with God," since ostensibly prayer can include listening. I don't like this answer for myself much either. First of all, I have never been so lucky as to hear a voice, in words, that I can name as the voice of God. Surely a divine power has ways of talking that go far beyond talk, and deeper. These days I'm thinking of prayer more as connection to the divine. Maybe more specifically, it is paying attention to the divine, or simply openness to the influence of the divine. It's like leaving the porch light on just in case someone wants to come over, even when no concrete invitations have yet been made. Or like holding my own tongue when conversing with a friend, so that there's enough space for their ideas—I won't hear them unless I can stop running my own mouth.

Somehow this way of defining prayer, as simply opening a channel of connection between myself and the divine, has helped me to spend much more time in prayer. I can do it even at times when I'm not sure about God or Jesus, at times when I don't have anything to say, and at times when I'm afraid to say what I would say. It takes the pressure off having the right words or the right intentions or my fear of being trite or silly or selfish. When I use the strategies in this chapter, sometimes the words I write are words I am saying *to* God, but other times they're words I'm just saying to clear the air, so that there's *room* for God should God choose to show up.

I went to a public high school in Texas in the late 1980s where every choir concert, football game—pretty much anything important—was preceded by group prayer. I always marveled how bold the sayers of these prayers seemed: they just out and asked God for things they wanted. I mean, sometimes little piddly stuff, like let us beat the Tigers, or help Brandon achieve a B– or better on his trig test so that he could remain eligible. Somehow, it never really took with me. I never could pray for myself. Wasn't God kind of busy with other people, the ones lacking clean water or finding out they had cancer or someone like that? With the more deserving people.

I also lived a long time without really praying in any wordful way. When I would be in church, and someone (many times me) would read aloud the Prayer of the Day or the Prayers of the People, I would read or listen to the words and try hard to feel them. Surely just saying words wasn't useful; I was supposed to be praising God, beseeching God. I was at least supposed to be *doing something*, right? Yet there I stood, most of the time drifting off somewhere around the second sentence or so. On a really good day, at least I'd find myself thinking a bit about my posture, grounding my feet into the floor and straightening my spine in a kind of meditative stance. At some point, I'd hear the other people mumble, "Amen," and I was off the hook.

My own prayers were and are usually silent meditations, like those moments standing in the pews noticing my posture, but with clearer intentions. I put my feet on the floor, slow myself down, and see what happens. A wise woman taught me how to put my hand on my heart and ask, "What do I know to be true?" Sometimes I can do that and learn something.

This was all fine until I became a scholar of writing and was convinced by the data and by my own nonprayer experiences that writing not only says things that we *say*, but it can tell us what we *mean* to say. We write our way *into* our ideas or *into* our beliefs just as much as we write *about* those things. And so I started to try journaling as prayer, starting in a letter-like, diary-like manner as I assumed was the way it was done. "Dear God," I'd begin, and then one of two things would happen. One, I couldn't really think what to say to God. Surely God already knows whatever it is, right? Or two, I might get writing, and the words and feelings would start coming, but I would realize somewhere on the second or third page that I'd sort of forgotten to address God and was talking to myself.

The way I think about this now is: exactly. God does know, if you believe in the kind of God who knows things. And what is writing really useful for, if any messages we might send to the divine are already known? Well, it's great for discovering what is in my mind and heart, and for reflecting on that. So, my uses of writing for prayer do sometimes include talking to God, but they also use writing as a way to plan for that talk, as a way to reflect on it, as a way of listening, and as a way of learning from what we might hear if we listen.

## A GLOW AND A GROW

A strategy I go to often comes straight out of the playbook of any elementary school teacher of writing: "a glow and a grow." Writing teachers use it as a frame for giving feedback to young writers, with the "glow" being something they're doing well and the "grow" being something to work on. I sometimes use it with my own children too, as a way of reflecting on their choices over a day or a week. Here, we use it to connect with the divine.

In one space, describe something that you're "glowing" about. It could be an accomplishment, something you're proud of, but it might also be something beautiful that you saw, something you appreciate, something you respond warmly to.

In the other space, identify an area in which you sense the need to grow. This may or may not be related to your "glow." This may be something you want to get better at or something you'd like to learn. Perhaps there's a mistake for which you'd like to make amends, or a hard feeling you're in that you'd like to move through. Use the "grow" space to think about that.

Sometimes the writing is more concrete; I remember writing about enjoying music (a glow) and wanting to expand by taking piano lessons (a grow). It seemed impossible to make this happen in the context of my busy life, but praying on it turned a vague wish into an intention. Whether my own or God's intention, I'm not sure. But I have now been taking piano lessons for six years, and what's more, the woman who teaches me has become a close friend who prays for me on the regular. Other times, the writing is more about spiritual growth. When I look closely at where I am and where I sense a need to grow and I ask God to help me, starting points appear.

Earlier in my life, when called upon to pray aloud, I have tended to end with a vague but well-meaning "and whatever your will." Which is a great stance to take, but in my own experience, it wasn't a great help in guiding me toward *what* is God's will. Glow/grow centers the prayer on finding out. For me, it's a way to begin by jumping in to the work of growing rather than standing at the side of the pool musing, "Hmm, I probably should get in there."

Glow

Grow

## FIVE FINGERS

Another issue that comes up for me is remembering or naming what is really on my mind when it comes time to pray. Or, a torrent of things is right at the surface, and I can't focus my intentions. I find this especially true when my focus in prayer is an area of worry or struggle: someone is sick, I have a problem, the world is unraveling. One way, truly, is simply to say, "God, fix it, please!" Or, if you want to get super spiritual, maybe close your eyes and meditate with that sentence as a kind of mantra: "GodfixitpleasepleasefixitpleaseGodpleasefixit." I have days where this is a beat pounding as sure as my heartbeat, I'll confess. I do think that this kind of prayer gives just as strong a connection to the divine as any other. But there's an argument for writing strategies that help slow me down in this stream of prayer—that help me make the abstract Big and Bad more concrete, with boundaries to hold it in place long enough to get quiet. This strategy helps me with finite, clear points of focus for prayer:

First, lay one of your hands on the paper and trace its outline with the other hand. (And if you're like me and you need to pause now and make a "hand turkey" just for old times' sake, I completely understand. Take all the time you need.)

Each of the fingers has space to note one point of concern. You can see my example below. Once I've got the fingers, I can't help but notice how each of mine is actually something in the *future* rather than a problem right now. Your mileage may vary, but for me this is the case at least half of the time. That is, I am worried about things that might happen, that I want to prevent happening, or that are going to happen and I simply don't know how they'll go. What if they go badly? So if you notice something all your "fingers" have in common, you're welcome.

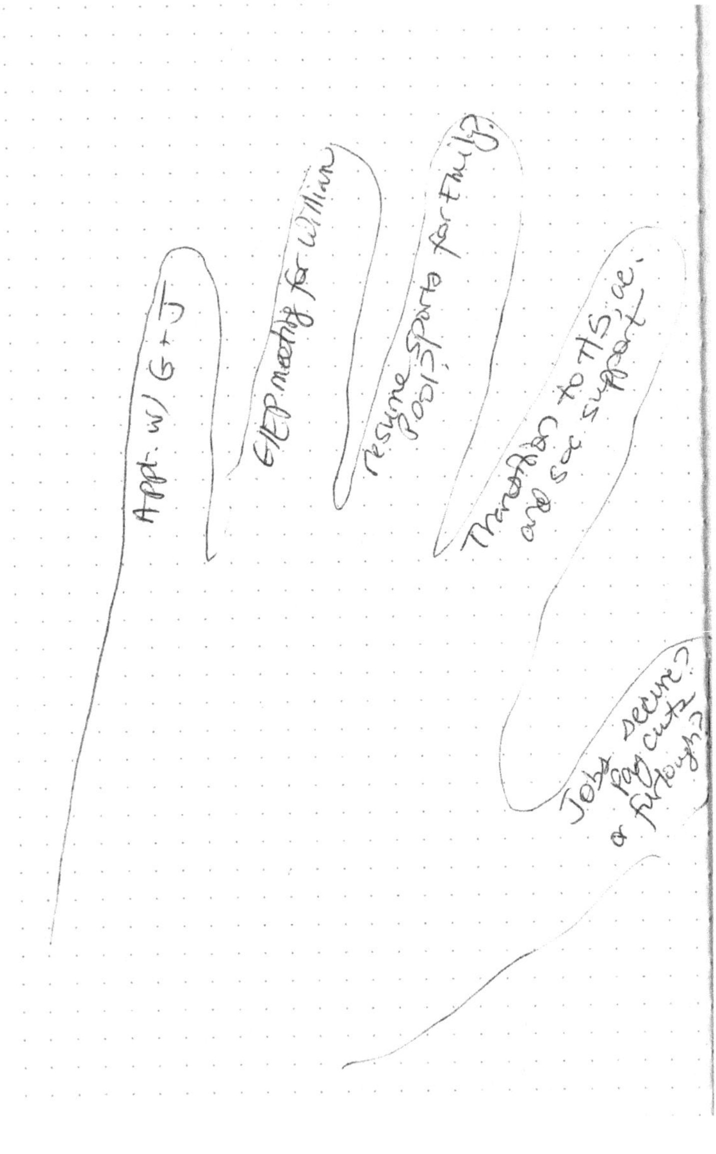

The next thing that I do and that I ask you to do, even if you feel stupid in the coffee shop or the airport or wherever you're working on this, is to touch each finger while you intentionally pray about that thing. Some people do this by touching the page. That works; tap your finger on the paper "finger" and pray it out, then move on to the next, and so on. I go one step further (overachiever, I know): I keep my eyes on the finger on the paper, but I use my other hand to touch the corresponding actual finger, gently tapping or even rubbing that finger. I have arthritis, so I'm usually unconsciously doing this anyway, to be fair, but there's a better reason also: the physical sensation keeps me much more focused. It's as though my worry, my desire to bring the worry to God, and my body and mind are all lined up, all doing the same thing at the same time. It's so rare that I'm like this; I'm one of those people with a brain that spins and spins if I'm not careful. Physically writing the words combined with physically connecting to those words as I talk to God about them reins me in somehow. It keeps God and me on the same page, literally.

So, I touch my finger and I look at the corresponding finger, and I speak aloud or silently and just "blab it out," as one of my students called it. I don't fashion a lovely petition; I unload. "OK, God, I'm worrying about my job—seems secure for now, but this is hard times like I've only read about, am I safe? I have not really saved enough to get by, and there's no way to get another job so I hope I'm safe . . . will there be salary cuts or furloughs? I hope not, don't feel like there's extra already . . ." It's embarrassing to put this down on paper in a book; it's like the scratches of a rat's feet on a wheel really, but that's the point: you're not putting it down on paper in a book or anywhere else that someone will read; you're using the five fingers as literal touchpoints to take it to God in a less-processed manner than that would be.

When you run out of gas on a finger, you just move to the next one. And when you're done, and the "blabbing" seems to have come to a stop, have a look at the center of that hand on the paper. First: God has us in God's hands. Maybe it's a cliché, but it's part of most every tradition: God is aware and God is there in hard moments. You might just rest there, thinking in a silent prayer how God is holding everything, how small each problem is in God's giant hand. Use imagery that makes sense for your tradition or your sense of God.

Second: You can place your fears gently, or throw them desperately, into divine hands. That is, you can take your own hand, the one that has been touching all this fear and worry, and transfer all you're holding into other hands, divine hands. When I do this, I sometimes place my palm back on the paper, imagining all the words I've said and feelings I've felt flowing back into the paper—into divine hands that can take it for a while or forever. I have also seen people ball their hand into a fist, then do a *fling* that opens the hand and throws the (imagined) stuff from their own hand into divine hands. There's no wrong way to do it; again, you're connecting verbally, nonverbally, emotionally, and physically to your sense of God here.

## VERSE FREEWRITE

Most of us have at some point tried to spend more time with the Bible, or with an important text from another tradition. Possibly you have succeeded in this, reading the Bible cover to cover in a year or gathering your family for a daily morning devotion or listening to Scripture as you work out. I have not.

Every now and then, what I do instead is go deep with some slice of Scripture using writing. Sometimes it's one I heard in a worship service and felt I needed more time to think through; sometimes it's one we'll consider in a class I've been asked to teach or a children's sermon I have been asked to preach. Once I've got a passage picked out, a series of steps that Peter Elbow calls "loop writing" helps me to go deeper.[1]

First, read the passage. When I gather people in workshops, I have them read it twice: First, I'll read it aloud, and you mark lines or phrases that really stand out. Then, you read it yourself, silently, also marking what stands out.

Second, choose a line or sentence or two that feels important. Maybe it feels like the passage's center of gravity. Maybe it is a line that most directly challenges your own existing point of view. Maybe it's one you feel you're not fully understanding. Copy that line at the top of your paper and read it again.

Now, under that line, spend five to ten minutes freewriting on that line. What strikes you about it? What does it help you to notice? What do you take it to be saying? There are no right answers here; you're simply trying to collect your impressions.

The next step is to read over what you have just written and highlight or circle a line that is especially interesting, that you could think more about. Copy it below, then write again. You can see an example from my own notebook below.

After five or ten minutes, again: choose a line of interest, copy it, then write again.

Keep on looping until you either run out of steam or have such a striking insight you can't go on. Did you realize something new about the meaning of the passage to you? About yourself or something in your life?

Philippians 4:6-7, 11-14, 8-9. Verse Freewrite

"Do not worry about anything, but in everything by prayer + supplication with thanksgiving let your requests be made known to God. And the peace of God, which surpasses all understanding, will guard your hearts + minds in Christ Jesus. . . (6-7)

I ~~[illegible]~~ have learned to be content with whatever I have. I know what it is to ~~[illegible]~~ have little and what it is to have plenty. In any and all circumstances I have learned the secret of ~~[illegible]~~ being well-fed + going hungry, of having plenty and being in need. I can do all things through him who strengthens me. (11-14)

Whatever ~~[illegible]~~ true, whatever is honorable, whatever is just, whatever is pure, whatever is pleasing, whatever is commendable, if there is any excellence, if there is anything worthy of praise, think about these things. Keep on doing the things you have learned + received + heard and seen in me, and the God of peace will be with you." (8-9)

I see so much about peace here. "The peace that surpasses all understanding. The God of peace. . . It doesn't say "God will fix it" or "God will fix you." Which is sometimes what I'm secretly expecting, even hoping God will do. God doesn't make it all better; God gives peace with what is. Is it a clue to how to activate this sense of peace:

"by prayer + supplication w/ thanksgiving let your requests be made known to God"

"think about these things" (the good and inspiring.)

And are they all "good things?" It doesn't actually say "think on sunshine and rainbows. It says think on truth, on justice, on what is excellent, right. these actually are not always pretty. It's that they're true and important. Not fluffy idealized clouds, ~~but~~ and in fact some are stormy clouds indeed. But I can picture these clouds clearing into TRUTH, and that by its nature is more peaceful.

Even a hard truth, when faced straight-on, can bring peace.

Even a hard truth, when faced straight on, can bring peace.

This is an idea that I'm placing a lot of faith in right now. I'm facing some pretty hard truths. They suck; they're things I wish weren't true. But, I already have felt a kind of peace in facing them, even when they don't get easier, problems not magically solved or anything.

Leslie has taught me this little practice of putting my hand on my heart, look into myself with kindness and ask "What do I know to be true?" And notice/listen what comes up. Most of the time there is a truth there. It's kind of weird to learn that after all these years of being a kind of seeker, always wanting to "get to the bottom" of things, that I was so un-used to looking inside for truth. How could I know anything? But it really does happen that I know sometimes. Right now this truth about J. and me is so hard. It activates all these paths of action that I have tried so hard not to take! And only sometimes do want to take. But once you see a truth, can you just go on how you were before you knew it? I can't, I want the peace of knowing what's true and living into the truth as best I can. It feels more peaceful somehow even though it means creating a lot of turbulence.

Once you see a truth, can you just go on how you were before you knew it?

I'm thinking of times I lived untruly — told myself stories about what was going on that were untrue, or kept a story intact by shutting out / ignoring / overlooking a truth. It is so hard. You have to squint through little cracks at your life, or twist your mind up into a tangled shape to make it happen. So I pretended that I hadn't seen things, or else that they didn't mean what they suggested. The times that I explained away something bad, or made something my own fault that wasn't, or said I was tired when I was sad, and so on.

I told myself stories.

What a capability of the mind this is! But unfortunately, a lot of times the story I had to tell myself was that I wouldn't / couldn't have better, that "kinda bad" was good enough.

It actually gets me all the way back to the verse from the beginning — "Whatever is good, whatever is true, and so on, think about these things." I've been trying to do this, but in a new + true way. Don't point myself toward unhappiness just thinking it's "right" or it's what I am supposed to do or thought I would do. Do the thing that is true. And how you know what is true (for me anyway) involves "thinking about these things." When I have a handle on what truth, good, justice actually look and feel like, I also have a better handle on what is not.

## CLUSTER PRAYER

Sometimes what we need is to streamline our thoughts and prayers, to make them more linear or more focused or to consider them one at a time. My mind tends to run fast, too fast, especially when I'm hurting or just especially excited, and it needs help containing a thought for long enough to understand it.

But our wild minds, our racing thoughts, our tangled stream of associations—this beautiful mess is real too, isn't it? And while sometimes we learn by untangling the threads, other times we learn from the connections that the tangles might reveal.

What's on your heart today? Jot it in the center oval. I'm a worrier, so mine tend to be things I'm anxious about. So, pretty much everything. You might name a person, an event, a decision, a situation. Once you've identified this focus, time to pray. As different aspects of your focus come to the front of your consciousness, jot them down as they occur to you, branching off the oval.

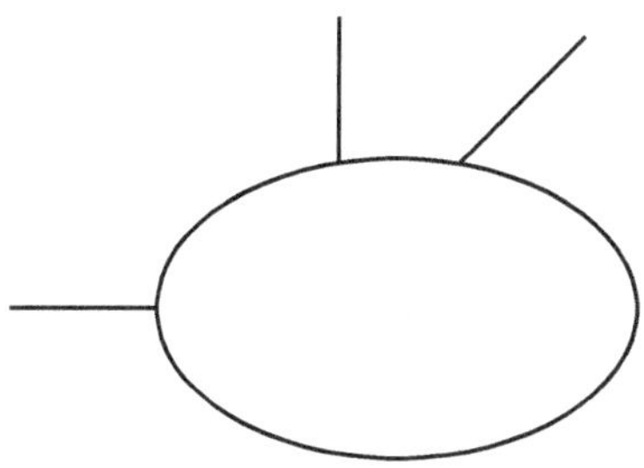

How long should you go on? This kind of question is the kind I'm always asking: unanswerable. One writing teacher friend answers kids who annoyingly ask her, "How long does it have to be?" with the even more annoying, "How long is a piece of string?" Or, my piano teacher friend Lauren, when I asked her how long I should practice, answered cryptically, "Keep going until something changes." I hated this advice, but it worked. With a tough passage, I play through it, using the strategies she suggested, until . . . it feels different. My brain has made some mind-hand connection it didn't have before. Or my eyes have come to recognize what this or that chord both sounds like and feels like, instead of me reading individual notes. I usually can't put my finger on it, but something has changed, and the piece of music is more my own.

So, keep going until something changes. Then say, "Amen."

Isn't that what prayer is like? If we get "answers," they're almost never words like "Yes," "No," or "Definitely quit that job." What I experience with prayer isn't about answers at all. It's about showing up, deciding that entering a shared space with God is something I am willing to do. It's about letting God use the time and the writing to show me something I hadn't realized. To name something I hadn't spoken. Or just to invite God into my self. When I do this, not every time but always over time, something changes.

# 6

# WRITE TO SURVIVE, WRITE TO THRIVE

## MAKING WRITING ROUTINE

Many of us come to writing—or to the idea of self-care overall—in times of emergency. That is, we pick up a pen when a transition occurs, when we face a decision, when we're in need. People give us blank notebooks for milestones like graduations, not "just because." I lived my life for many years with an "if it ain't broke, don't fix it" attitude. No check-ups, just urgent care. No prevention, just patch jobs. I'm not kidding—I drove a car without maintenance for so long it eventually cracked a head, and way more times than I can count, I've worked so hard and long to meet an unrealistic goal that I then had to collapse for days or weeks afterward. Am I the only one here who can sit at my desk so long I forget to go to the bathroom?

Writing for self-care, however, works best if we treat it like maintenance, not repair. Brushing your teeth is better than fillings or dentures; changing your oil is better than replacing your car; daily exercise is better than going from couch to marathon. If, as a flawed human being, always both a sinner and a saint, I am always in need of ongoing spiritual restoration, then it seems to me I should also be always engaged in the work of examination and reflection, no?

The main concern I hear from writers in classes and workshops is "I don't have time." I understand this—as a scholar, as a single mom, as a chronic overcommitter, and honestly, just as an American in the current era—I always feel as though I'm short on time. I've named this state of mind "the behind feeling." When the behind feeling is strong, I feel I'm behind from before I wake up each morning until I've fallen asleep each evening. It's a terrible way to live.

I'll tell you what a loving but tough mentor told me: you have time, you're just choosing to spend it on something else. When he said this to me initially, I'll confess I was deeply offended. I was at that time a beginning scholar overwhelmed by my career and a needy young baby, new in town with no network of support and not enough money for help. My house was piled with dirty laundry, I wasn't getting enough sleep, I owed work all over the place, and I needed a haircut. Who was this older man, who had enjoyed a stay-at-home wife when his own kids were young, to tell me how much time I had? But I came to see what he meant one evening when, as I often did, I sat down after putting the baby to bed with a laptop and my cold, half-eaten dinner, aiming to grade just a few more papers or finish that late book review. I was choosing to open that laptop, which meant I was choosing to spend that time doing work (slowly and poorly, since by then I was too tired to think well at all) instead of watching TV, or cleaning the kitchen, or taking a bath, or writing in my notebook. I could choose differently. Of course there are limits to this—if I don't sometimes choose to do work, I'll lose my job, and if I don't sometimes choose to clean the kitchen, I'll breed disease. But each time, it's a choice, and each time something else can be chosen. As that mentor said later on, when you really want to do something, chances are you'll let some other things go. And of course I couldn't and wouldn't let caring for my daughter go, or making dinner, or living in a clean home, or succeeding moderately in my job go: All of these things were important to me. But, they weren't all *equally* important *every* time. I can assess what is important in a given moment in time and choose accordingly. And for my soul to be in anything like good health, I will have to choose that it is important at least sometimes. More than never, which was my previous record on that choice. There have to be some moments in which I matter most, or failing that, in which connecting to God in my life matters most.

Scan your life for open moments. In fact, better not to look for "open" moments. You've already filled them with something. Look instead for moments of choice. You might even turn back to the time log you made back in chapter 3 and see if any pop out at you there.

Here are some moments in which writers in my classes, retreats, writing groups, and friend group have found they can choose to write. I promise you they are as busy as you or I are; the key is that they identified moments where a choice was possible, and then they either dropped the activity they had previously chosen, completed that activity in a different, faster way, or found a different time for that activity. They chose writing:

- In the first five or ten minutes of the day, over coffee, before waking the children for school

- In five to ten quiet minutes in the church sanctuary before worship began
- During the commercials on an evening TV show
- On the closed toilet seat while her young son played in the tub
- In the office for the first five or ten minutes after arriving, before turning on the computer
- While waiting for many, many medical appointments during a bout with cancer
- In the car while his wife drove the family on vacation
- In the car via voice recording, while driving (this works in a different way than physically writing, and it may not invoke the exact same benefits as shown in the research, but it's much better than nothing at all)
- On the fifteen-minute break between evening college classes
- While the casserole (or fish sticks, or frozen pizza) is in the oven

I don't think these writers are less busy than we are. And they're not more spiritual either. They simply decided to try it. Then they decided again. And again.

To make the decision to write easier to make, you may need to alter your environment for success. You wouldn't practice your musical instrument in a noisy room full of people speaking to you. To make writing easier to choose, try to have pen and paper wherever you are going to be. For me, this means a small notebook in my purse, another in my work bag, and one more in my car. Jot a couple of the activities from this book into a page near the back of your notebook, so you're never without an idea to write about (or heck, buy multiple copies for all of the places you frequent!). Try making a date with a friend for writing—Phoebe and I meet for about an hour of coffee, chatting, writing, and optional sharing. Identify a cue for writing somewhere in your day: Is it the coffee machine beeping to tell you it's ready? Is it right after you've taken the dog out in the evening? Is it Thursday nights when you wait for your kid at karate? Is it in bed when you used to watch TV?

## WRITING AS A MINDFUL SPIRITUAL PRACTICE

In her lovely book of advice to writers, *Writing Down the Bones*, Natalie Goldberg explains that "Writers live twice," going along with our regular lives while also holding certain thoughts and details in mind to relive/write about later.[1]

This is one of my favorite things about writing: It can stop time. That is, when writing, I'm only writing. I'm looking only at a subject I am writing about and at myself in the act of writing it. And the more time we have with any subject, including ourselves, the more opportunity to understand it. In the act of writing, I notice more. Things aren't going by in my mind or before me quite so quickly. I am limited a bit by the speed of my hand and by the need to be articulating at the same time I am remembering or observing. My body and my mind are doing the same thing—unusual for a person like me whose head tends to race into the future.

In this way, writing can be seen as a mindfulness practice.

Sometimes people think of mindfulness as a brain completely empty of thought; feeling this to be impossible, they either reject mindfulness as a goal or claim they are not good at meditating. I am one of the latter—truly, my mind doesn't get very empty, and what it's filled with isn't always top quality either. But the term is mind*full*, not mind*less*. That is, to be mindful is to be more aware of and less automatic about what is in there, not to ignore it. The question in mindfulness—and in spiritual writing—is something like, "What is within and around me? What is, what could be?" The storytelling that opened our writing work in chapter 2 reveals not only that we make stories of everything but also *that these stories can be revised*. The noticing that characterizes chapter 3 is mindfulness practice in that it helps to become aware of where and how we are, making visible what is usually present yet invisible to us. The writing we use for discernment in chapter 4 is less mindful in the sense that it tends to be oriented toward the future, which doesn't yet exist, but it does represent mindful practice in that it asks us to notice what we imagine, think, and feel *now* as we contemplate various future paths. And of course I am not alone in saying that prayer is a mindful practice. It's mindful practice that informs the statement at the beginning of this chapter that "the writer lives twice."

I'll confess that even as a scholar who literally spends my days researching and teaching writing, and even as someone who has kept some kind of notebook or journal most of my life, I really never understood diaries. That is, the basic diary that, true to its name, contains a daily account of someone's activities sounded to me like a huge waste of time. It was actually this thought, that an account of my days would be horribly boring, that stopped me from all of my attempts at diary-keeping, even in those coveted gift diaries with a tiny lock and a tiny pen. Who would want to read about a day in which I ate a couple of meals, did some chores, got the mail, and watched TV? Surely the people in later generations will have better things to read. It's only as an adult and after a lot of learning, I'll admit, that I came to see that we're not just writing to produce an account. Nobody wants to read that list of what I did in a boring day, and no one needs to read it. It's what those notes and memories mean to *us* that matters. The value isn't in the document to be produced; it's in the thinking, feeling, and reflection that occur in the production of the document. That is, the process. It's not about the poem or novel or short story you'll write (for the public) someday; it's about writing itself as an activity. When we write not just to record but to reflect, we open ourselves to spiritual learning.

It's worth saying as well that to reflect on anything, some mindfulness is required. To move through remembering, describing, and acting on experiences,[2] we must call those experiences into mind and then hold them there for further processing: to describe them (such as in writing), to plan actions, and then to bring them with us into future action. It's a way of paying attention to what has happened, taking it seriously, and letting it change or confirm our course, whether in doing, in thinking, or perhaps in relating to others. It's a kind of attention that honors our own capacity as learners.

For Christians, and for many other faith traditions, walking with God leads to transformation. In this book, I have tried to describe and to model the ways that writing, too, provokes transformation, and how writing and faith can work together for us to take better care of our spiritual selves. Ultimately, self-care, and writing as a practice of self-care, go beyond helping with stress, fear, distraction, and burnout in the short term to something greater and longer lasting. Writing can help us thrive.

# Appendix

## Writing with Others: Some Notes for Leaders

All of the activities in this book can be and have been used with groups in classes, retreats, and workshops. This section offers advice for adapting the activities, making them interactive for groups, and supporting writers as they work. But first, I want to lay out some key ideas for informal writing and sharing that draw on my experience as a writing researcher and practitioner in this area. They won't be surprising to anyone who leads small groups regularly, but they're worth articulating because adding writing adds some special sensitivities. I offer them here as things to do *before* your group meets, *during* shared writing time, and *after* the session is over.

### BEFORE:

#### Help people know there's no wrong way

First and foremost, it is important to remember that many people are fearful about writing or sharing their writing. This is usually based on negative past experiences with writing in school, but it is also linked to a common feeling that "my writing is me." Differences in writing speed, writing apprehension, correctness in writing, and writing confidence all link to differences in educational opportunities, age, and people's sense of themselves as smart or capable. We want to signal, first and foremost, that all writing will be valuable and that no writing will be shared without the writer's decision to do so.

Many people are also fearful about sharing spiritual reflection. Sometimes they have had previous negative experiences doing so. I remember becoming reluctant after I remarked once in a Bible study that the fishermen seemed irresponsible when dropping their nets to follow Jesus (those things were expensive!) to a reaction somewhere between "duh" and stunned silence from others in the room. It was years before I spoke aloud about Scripture again. Others may have concern that the things they say about God might be somehow accidentally heretical or will reflect a lack of knowledge about Scripture or theology. In my adult Sunday school—which I even coteach!—almost everyone around the table has way more Bible knowledge than I do. It can feel intimidating.

### Remember the purpose of the gathering

This is why our primary goal in all interactions related to the writing in this book must be to validate and support participants *simply for engaging in the work*. There is no need to respond to the writing as writing; its purpose is not to reach an audience but to help the writer. As long as it is doing that, it's good writing for its purpose. And I feel strongly that there is also no need to respond to any spiritual content with information, correction, or advice about God or spiritual matters, because again, receiving another person's perspective or making beliefs more orthodox is not the purpose of this writing. The few exceptions I have seen to this have all had something in common: The writer asked for it. That is, if you are a faith leader and this person has asked you a question, or this person has asked you for help, then of course you're going to answer or help. But you'll do it lovingly, understanding that the writer asking is asking from a place of need rather than one of curiosity or some educational interest.

## DURING:

### Write along with the group

Just because you're the group leader doesn't mean you're not also a writer. I've done each of these activities dozens of times (and sometimes more!) with groups of all kinds, and I always still find more and new things to discover each time I approach them. When you sit back and supervise while participants write, you seem like a teacher. When you jump in to write and share alongside the others, you seem like a teacher or leader but also like a human being with a spiritual life and life story of your own. You also get a precious set of chances to model the attitudes and behavior you'd like to see in all the members. You get a clearer sense of how much time tasks take and how tiring or difficult they are. Finally, you get empathy—which stops you from making the mistake of asking participants to do something you won't or can't do for yourself.

### Offer multiple ways of sharing

I usually offer that the best and easiest way to share is simply to read aloud what you have written. Just hearing yourself read it will open up new thinking, often. But at times people don't feel ready to share, or are afraid of being judged, or choose not to share out of existing relationships with someone in the room. That's all OK. What I say is something like this:

"Most of you will want to just read what you have. Hear yourself say the words, and let your partner experience the words as you wrote them, fresh and unpolished. But if what you've written feels too raw or unsafe to share, or for some reason you just feel strongly about not sharing it, that's fine. Perhaps you can tell about it instead of reading it. Or perhaps you can read part but not all. If you need to, you can just be an extraloving listener, and know that we are here for you in whatever you're working through."

When people are married or related to each other, as they might be in some congregational settings, I also take care to mix up the groups so that relatives and loved ones are not always grouped together.

### Help participants develop shared commitments

Anything you can do to grease the social wheels for your writers, do it. Food is never a bad idea.

Take some time to talk about ground rules. These are the things that matter in most every kind of group: clear time management, monitoring individuals' airtime to ensure all get a turn, honoring privacy and discretion, and so on. I've also found that it's best to make sure group participants also buy into these commitments, so rather than naming them all myself, I open the process up and let members contribute their "rules" in their own words.

## Protect your writers

If you have people writing and sharing from personal experiences and feelings, you're responsible for making sure the environment is a safe place to do so. One way I work to achieve this is by telling hard stories about myself and reading direct, raw pieces right out of my own notebook before asking others to do the same. When they respond to me gently (as they always do), I pause and point it out, naming the gentle ways I would like them to respond to others as well.

That said, often there is someone in the group who likes to explain and inform. And often, those explanations and points of information tend to flow "downstream" through status or power relationships: men explaining to women; older explaining to younger; members of dominant groups explaining to members of historically disempowered groups. It's not helpful, and it's often hurtful. When this happens in my own groups, I am ready to respond gently but firmly with language like:

"I'm mindful of the time, so I want to move on to someone else."

"Remember why we're here. We want all writers to be heard equally."

"That's one thought. Does someone else have a different thought?"

These cues are usually enough. But I have also been known to grab someone in the hall for a second and say, "Hey, thanks so much for that point. The thing is, not everyone feels so comfortable, so can you watch your airtime?"

But. If they're airing out racism or misogyny or other trash, I do have to call it out right there. Immediately. For instance,

I'll say, "Our group will not work unless everyone is safe. That statement is not OK with me."

### Help participants know how to respond

The goal in responding to the kind of writing we're doing is not to improve it; it is to help its author feel heard and known while engaging in the sometimes-tough task of getting to know themselves. So, it's important that feedback be specific and noncorrective. Here are some examples of language to use (and to teach participants):

Thank you for sharing that.
When you read that, I felt ____
That sounds really hard/fulfilling/scary/joyful/etc.
I love how _______
What kind of response would help you right now?
(Often people will say "no response." Make sure they know about this option.)

Model this yourself, always. People really will follow your lead. Post these phrases on a whiteboard or share on a handout. Then, eavesdrop on the group while they share so that you can notice and redirect anything that's veering toward critique. That's not what this work is about.

## AFTER:

How will you follow up? Of course many people give some kind of evaluation afterward, and that isn't a bad idea. But I also tend to simply ask if a group or any of its members would like to keep going. I can't facilitate dozens of ongoing groups myself, though, so what I do is offer to meet with them—briefly right then and there, or at a later date, depending on how much energy seems appropriate for me and for them. In a brief meeting, I'll prompt them to get multiple dates on the calendar and to choose some ground rules for what they'll bring (some like to write ahead of time and meet to talk, while others meet to write in shared quiet and then talk immediately). They don't need me.

Don't forget to reflect on yourself as a leader. When did you sense the deepest engagement? Disengagement? When did things feel excited and fast, or slow and deep, or just boring? Can you recall something specific from each participant (this is something I practice so that I better focus on listening well in a session rather than jumping on to the next thing)?

# Notes

## Chapter 1


1 Sultan, N. Embodied self-care: Enhancing awareness and acceptance through mindfulness-oriented expressive writing self-disclosure. *J. Creat. Ment. Health* **13**, 76–91 (2018).

2 Brody, L. R. & Park, S. H. Narratives, Mindfulness, and the Implicit Audience. *Clin. Psychol. Sci. Pract.* **11**, 147–154 (2004).

3 Poon, A. & Danoff-Burg, S. Mindfulness as a moderator in expressive writing. *J. Clin. Psychol.* **67**, 881–895 (2011).

4 Pennebaker, J. W. *Opening Up: The Healing Power of Expressing Emotions*. (Guilford Press, 1990).

5 Pennebaker, J. W. *Emotion, Disclosure and Health*. (American Psychological Association, 2002).

6 Pennebaker, J. W. Writing about Emotional Experiences as a Therapeutic Process. *Psychol. Sci.* **8**, 162–166 (1997).

7 Pennebaker, J. & Evans, J. *Expressive Writing: Words That Heal.* (Idyll Arbor, 2014).

8 Pennebaker, J. W. & Smyth, J. M. *Opening Up by Writing It Down, Third Edition: How Expressive Writing Improves Health and Eases Emotional Pain*. (Guilford, 2017).

9 *Boud, D. Reflection: Turning Experience into* Learning. (Routledge Falmer, 1985).

10 Whitney, A. E., McCracken, C., & Washell, D. *Teaching Writers to Reflect: Strategies for a More Thoughtful Writing Workshop*. (Heinemann, 2019).

## Chapter 2

1 Frank, C. Mapping Our Stories: Teachers' Reflections on Themselves as Writers. *Lang. Arts* **80**, 185–195 (2003).
2 Blau, S. *The Literature Workshop: Teaching Texts and Their Readers.* (Heinemann, 2003).
3 Elbow, P. *Writing without Teachers.* (Oxford University Press, USA, 1998).

## Chapter 3

1 Robinson, J. P. Americans Less Rushed but No Happier: 1965–2010 Trends in Subjective Time and Happiness. *Soc. Indic. Res.* **113**, 1091–1104 (2013).
2 Robinson, J. P. & Tracy, E. A Less Stressed, Less Harried—and Slightly Happier—America. *Contexts* **15**, 74–76 (2016).
3 Newman, K. Why You Never Seem to Have Enough Time. *Greater Good; Greater Good Science Center at UC Berkeley* https://greatergood.berkeley.edu/article/item/why_you_never_seem_to_have_enough_time (2019).
4 Docter, P. *Inside Out.* (Pixar Animation Studio, Walt Disney Studios Motion Pictures, 2015).
5 Plutchik, R. A psychoevolutionary theory of emotions. *Soc. Sci. Inf.* **21**, 529–553 (1982).
6 Tweed, J. How to Use the Wheel of Emotions to Write Better Fictional Characters. *Medium* https://medium.com/swlh/how-to-use-the-wheel-of-emotions-to-write-better-fictional-characters-a86ba6381fe2 (2019).
7 Smith, L. B. *Unsent Letters: Writing to Resolve and Renew.* (Walking Stick Press, 2002).

## Chapter 4

1 Bolton, G. *Writing Routes: A Resource Handbook of Therapeutic Writing*. (Jessica Kingsley Publishers, 2011).
2 Whitney, A. E. Writer, Teacher, Person: Tensions between Personal and Professional Writing in a National Writing Project Summer Institute. *Engl. Educ.* **41**, 235–258 (2009).
3 Tierney, J. Do You Suffer from Decision Fatigue?—The New York Times. *New York Times Magazine* (2011).

## Chapter 5

1 Elbow, P. *Writing with Power: Techniques for Mastering the Writing Process*. (Oxford University Press, 1998).

## Chapter 6

1 Goldberg, N. *Writing Down the Bones: Freeing the Writer Within, 2nd Edition*. (Shambhala, 2005).
2 Kabat-Zinn, J. Getting Started with Mindfulness. *Mindful* https://www.mindful.org/meditation/mindfulness-getting-started/ (2020).